Migraine and its Variants

Cover illustration: Drawing of a stone carving on the Bell Tower of New College, Oxford. This may depict a person with migraine holding his head and shielding his eyes.

Migraine and its Variants

by

George Selby

MD, FRCP (London), FRCP (Edinburgh), FRACP
Visiting Neurologist, Royal North Shore Hospital, Sydney

ADIS Health Science Press
Sydney • Auckland • Bristol • Boston • Hong Kong • Tokyo

Migraine and its Variants

National Library of Australia
Cataloguing-in-Publication entry

Selby, George.
  Migraine and its variants.

  Bibliography.
  Includes index.
  ISBN 0 86792 015 7.

  1. Migraine.   2. Headache.   I. Title.

616.8'57

ADIS Health Science Press
404 Sydney Road, Balgowlah, NSW 2093, Australia

Foreword

Migraine has been known for thousands of years, judging from symptoms recorded in literature. In fact the term arose from the writings of Galen in the second century A.D. In modern medical literature the clinical features of common, classic, and complicated migraine and those of cluster headache are well documented and more or less agreed upon by medical investigators. Although physicians now understand these conditions descriptively and investigators have measured many concomitant physiological and biochemical changes, the pathophysiological mechanism of migraine has still escaped us.

Dr George Selby is a distinguished neurologist and a past president of the Australian Association of Neurologists. He is recognized by his colleagues as a perceptive clinician and a stimulating teacher. His forte is careful management of patients. He has taken a special interest in observing and treating patients with migraine for thirty years or more and has recorded many of his observations in the medical literature.

In this book, Doctor Selby presents a succinct and practical approach to the understanding of migraine and migraine variants and their management. The clinical descriptions are concise and clear and he presents an excellent review of the mechanisms of headache that have been espoused by a variety of authors. He reviews available treatment programs for each type of migraine from the standpoint of prophylaxis and treatment of the individual headache. This includes an unbiased description of the possible relationship of allergens to migraine and the role of other environmental stimuli.

This book will provide medical practitioners with an understanding of migraine and will provide them with a practical and safe approach to management of their patients with migraine.

Jack P. Whisnant, M.D.
Professor of Neurology
Mayo Clinic and Mayo Medical School
Rochester, Minnesota, U.S.A.

Preface

Pain is the most common symptom for which the primary physician is consulted and pain in the head occurs more frequently than in any other part of the body. The head has special importance in the body image of mankind, because it contains the seat of our intellect, thoughts and emotions. It is therefore not surprising that pain in the head may create concern out of proportion to its severity and significance.

About one in every five patients referred to the specialist neurologist suffers from headache; the majority have migraine. This reflects not only the prevalence of migraine and the concern it creates in the sufferer; it is also an indication of inadequate therapeutic results and of physicians' feelings of insecurity that they may have overlooked a more sinister intracranial lesion. Advances in technology have provided us with reliable diagnostic tools ranging from electroencephalography to brain scanning by computerized axial tomography, but the enormous cost of such investigations is now arousing the criticism of governments and of society. There are increasing demands that the physician must show concern for the public purse as well as for the patient's welfare.

It is the aim of this book to provide family physicians with guidelines which may help them recognize clinical criteria which justify special investigations. Some of the enormous literature on experimental work searching for the cause and mechanism of migraine headache will be reviewed briefly, but the book is not intended as a scientific treatise.

The clinical study of every patient with migraine has many rewards. We have the opportunity to witness transient focal disturbances of cerebral function due to changes in the calibre of intracranial and extracranial arteries and we will see a spectrum of dysfunction of the autonomic nervous system. Migraine provides us with an almost unique opportunity to study the relationship between genetic traits, personality structure and environmental and emotional circumstances in the causation of disease.

Research in recent years has made great strides and has drawn attention to specific biochemical events which can influence arterial calibre and contribute to migraine, but the gaps are still much wider than the extent of our knowledge. This book is, therefore, written with humility and awareness of our ignorance of the protean causes of migraine; it will raise more questions than it answers. It is published in the hope that it will stimulate renewed interest in the subject and so contribute to the better management of the patient with the limited therapeutic armamentarium at our disposal.

George Selby
Sydney, October 1982

Acknowledgements

This book could never have been written without the help of my wife, Deirdre. She did not complain about the many days devoted to writing rather than to more relaxing pursuits; she searched for the most suitable case histories from my files, she typed and checked the manuscript and prepared the bibliography.

My sincere thanks are due to Dr Peter M. Williamson, who permitted me to use the case histories of some of his patients and to Professor Mervyn Eadie for constructive advice on the manuscript and for providing valuable information on pharmacological aspects of the treatment of migraine.

I am particularly grateful to Professor Jack P. Whisnant for writing the foreword and for his helpful comments on several topics discussed in the book.

It is a pleasure to thank Mr Richard Drew and the Department of Medical Illustration of the Royal North Shore Hospital of Sydney for preparing the drawings and illustrations. I wish to express my gratitude to Mr Tom MacLennan and to Ms Pamela Petty of Adis Health Science Press for their patience, courtesy and help.

I am indebted to Oxford University Press, New York, for permission to publish an illustration from *Headache and Other Head Pain*, 2nd Edition, by Harold G. Wolff on page 249 and to Professor William F. Hoyt and to the Williams and Wilkins Company, Baltimore, for permission to publish an illustration from *Clinical Neuro-Ophthalmology*, Vol. 2, 3rd Edition, by F.B. Walsh and W.F. Hoyt on page 1663.

Contents

Chapter 1

General Introduction

Historical Review

Migraine is probably as old as mankind. The earliest description of headache associated with visual symptoms is attributed to a Sumerian writer 3000 years before Christ (Garrison, 1969). In the second half of the First Century AD, Aretaeus of Cappadocia (AD 30-90) defined heterocrania as a pain involving either the entire cranium or its right or left half separately. During the Second Century AD, Galen (AD 138-201) was the first to use the term hemicrania, which was later corrupted to hemigranea and from this "megrim" and migraine were derived (Dalessio, 1968). Galen was concerned about the nausea and vomiting which accompanied hemicrania and postulated a sympathetic connecting system between the stomach and the brain. In accordance with the humoral hypotheses prevailing at his time, he believed that bile and other harmful substances were the cause of headache. The next detailed description of migraine was written by Avicenna almost a thousand years later. Though not a medical scientist, Hildegard of Bingen (1098-1180), a nun and mystic who suffered from severe migraine, left two manuscript codices (cited by Sacks, 1971) which contain a vivid account and illustrations of brilliant, luminous and coloured visions which were undoubtedly migrainous. Practitioners of the art of healing were evidently content to accept the dogma of older writers for the next 600 years until Thomas Willis (1621-1675) first drew attention to vascular factors in the genesis of headache without entirely abandoning the humoral hypotheses. He refers to dilatation of blood vessels and obstructions to the flow of blood and exhorts the sufferers to abstain from exercise, baths and wine.

In the 18th Century, the detailed autobiographical writings of Lepois (1714) and the observations and studies published by Wepfer (1787) in Germany and by Tissot (1784) in France show a reawakening of interest in the causation and clinical features of migraine. Wepfer favoured the importance of vascular stasis and of changes in the calibre of cranial vessels while Tissot gave greater emphasis to the stomach and intestinal tract for the pathogenesis of migraine. During the late 18th and 19th Centuries the most lucid clinical descriptions of migraine and new theories of its causation were provided by physicians who themselves suffered from the disease, including Fothergill, Parry and DuBois-Reymond. Liveing (1873) wrote the first systematic account of migraine, *On Megrim, Sick Headache and some Allied Disorders: A Contribution to the Pathology of Nerve-Storms.* He thought that migraine was a familial allergy, recognized the many varieties of its clinical presentation and discussed the relationship of migraine to other paroxysmal disorders.

Gowers' classic *Manual of Diseases of the Nervous System,* (1893) devotes 20 pages to a detailed and erudite description of the clinical features of migraine, which can hardly be surpassed today. He recognized the importance of heredity in aetiology and considers a possible genetic relationship between migraine and epilepsy. Such a relationship was also postulated by Hughlings Jackson (1888) who stated that there is a "discharging lesion" of some part of the cerebral cortex in migraine as in epilepsy.

During the early years of this century many unproven and unscientific theories for the causation of migraine were published, which implicated "irritative forces" in the eyes, in the pituitary and other endocrine glands and again in the gut. The classic article on the mechanism of migraine headache and the action of ergotamine tartrate, published by Graham and Wolff in 1938, put an end to this era of unscientific confusion. During the last 40 years the literature on migraine has assumed vast proportions. The importance of genetic, constitutional and environmental factors, and of hormonal and biochemical changes contributing to alterations in the calibre of both intracranial and extracranial arteries are now receiving close scrutiny.

The reader interested in the history of migraine and in the evolution of scientific thought on this topic will find further details in the references of original work cited in this chapter.

Definition and Classification of Migraine

The great variety of aetiological factors and of clinical features of the migraine syndrome creates difficulties in any attempt at precise definition. The Research Group on Migraine and Headache of the World Federation of Neurology agreed on the following definition in 1969:

A familial disorder characterised by recurrent attacks of headache widely variable in intensity, frequency and duration. Attacks are commonly unilateral and are usually associated with anorexia, nausea and vomiting. In some cases they are preceded by, or associated with, neurological and mood disturbances. All the above characteristics are not necessarily present in each attack or in each patient. *(Hemicrania,* 1969).

This broad definition emphasises the essential paroxysmal nature of the syndrome and allows for the wide variations of the clinical spectrum, not only between individual patients, but also during the lifespan of a single sufferer.

An Ad Hoc Committee on Classification of Headache of the National Institute of Neurological Diseases and Blindness (1962) published a similar definition of "Vascular Headache of Migraine Type" and listed five particular varieties of headache, each sharing some, but not necessarily all, of the common features:

1. Classic migraine.
2. Common migraine.
3. Cluster headache, previously also called ciliary or migrainous neuralgia, or histamine cephalalgia.
4. Hemiplegic migraine and ophthalmoplegic migraine, which have been termed "complicated migraine" or *migraine accompagnée* in Continental literature.
5. Lower half headache.

This classification makes no specific reference to basilar migraine or to migraine syncope, which may be included under the heading of classic migraine. It is important to realise that an individual may suffer from more than one type of migraine; many patients have both classic and common migraine. This serves to illustrate the common aetiology and the experimental and clinical evidence that the same vascular, autonomic and biochemical mechanisms are involved in the genesis of all varieties of the migraine syndrome. The classification is concerned only with the clinical features which distinguish one type of migraine from another. These are described in detail in Chapter 4.

Prevalence and Incidence

It is not possible to compile accurate epidemiological data for the prevalence of migraine in a community. The difficulties are compounded from a lack of generally accepted diagnostic criteria and from the fact that probably no more than half the number of sufferers consult a doctor. It is not unusual to elicit a past history of migraine for which no advice was sought from a patient referred for investigation of some other neurological disease. Therefore, many of the published prevalence data probably underestimate the real frequency of migraine. Prevalence estimates derived from family practitioners (primary physicians) in the USA, UK and Scandinavia range from 0.5% to 20% of the population (Wolff, 1963; Refsum, 1968; Lance, 1970; Office of Health Economics, London, 1972). There is evidence that the prevalence of migraine increases from 1% at the age of 6 years to 5% at the age of 11 years (Bille, 1962); in males, the prevalence probably remains in the vicinity of 5% to 10% during adult life, but it increases to approximately 20% in women during the reproductive period. In both sexes the number of persons affected by migraine declines with advancing age, but statistics of incidence in people over 50 years of age are not available. From the data summarized above, we may estimate that from 5% to 10% of the community suffers from migraine or one of its variants at some time during their lives. As this would account for some 10 to 20 million people in the USA alone, migraine represents a major health problem.

It is even more difficult to get valid statistics of the amount of time lost from work because of migraine. The economic impact of this common illness is reduced by the high incidence in women of child-bearing age who receive no salary for their labours in the home, but suffer their misery in silence and make up for the temporary neglect of their domestic responsibilities on headache-free days. In a series of 104 migrainous factory workers, each of the men lost less than one day and the women a mean of 2.4 days per year because of migraine (Childs and Sweetnam, 1961).

It was thought that migraine is mainly a disease of intelligent individuals and of those belonging to higher social strata. However, data derived from the records of family and specialist physicians are not typical of all migraine sufferers. They take no account of the fact that persons in the higher social and professional classes are more prone and able to seek medical advice. More broadly based epidemiological studies have demonstrated that migraine may affect people of all social classes and that the disease is not directly influenced by intelligence levels.

Although there is general agreement that migraine is more common in women, an accurate estimate of sex incidence is not available. Kinnier Wilson (1940) found a female preponderance of 71.6% in 3278 cases of migraine summarized from 13 published series. In a series of 500 cases (Selby and Lance, 1960) 60% of patients were women and in a later series of 500 cases reported by Lance and Anthony (1966) the proportion of women patients was 75%. Some of these differences in sex incidence can be accounted for by the different age distribution of patients in reported series of cases. The peak incidence of migraine is in women during their reproductive years and then it is thought to be as high as 20% to 25%.

Age of Onset

The first attack of migraine occurs before the age of 40 years in at least 90% of patients. It is rare for migraine to begin after the age of 60 years. In women the highest incidence is between the ages of 25 and 45 years, while in men the age incidence does not vary between the ages of 20 and 65 years (Brewis *et al.,* 1966). In 500 patients studied by Selby and Lance (1960), the first attack of migraine was experienced before the age of 10 years in 21%; other authors have reported proportions of patients with onset of migraine during the first decade of life ranging from 12% (Krayenbühl and Heyck, 1955) to 30% (Balyeat and Rinkel, 1931). In a study of almost 9000 Swedish school children, aged from 7 to 15 years, 4% suffered from migraine (Bille, 1962).

Frequency of Attacks

Accurate figures of the frequency of migraine paroxysms are even more difficult to obtain than estimates of prevalence in a community or of sex and age incidence. Even in the individual patient the frequency of attacks will vary with age and with exposure to stresses and other precipitating factors in the environment. The source of the data may produce different results, because a neurological clinic or specialist will deal with more patients suffering from severe and frequent migraine than will a family physician.

From figures derived both from family physicians and specialist neurological clinics, we can estimate that about 15% of migraine sufferers will average one or more headaches per month at some stage of their lives. In the series of 500 patients attending a neurology clinic reviewed by Selby and Lance (1960), more than half reported from one to four attacks each month. In the 15% of patients in the same series who suffered more than 10 attacks a month, emotional triggers became increasingly important; some of the patients were unable to distinguish between true migraine and psychogenic tension headaches. The frequency of attacks tends to decline with advancing age. This may be due partly to a lower exposure to environmental precipitants and largely to the diminished elasticity of both intracranial and extracranial arteries which are no longer able to constrict or dilate as readily as they did during youth.

Economic Impact of Migraine

If we consider the high prevalence of migraine in the community and the frequency of recurring attacks in these patients, it becomes clear that this disease is a major drain on health expenditure, including the cost of both medical and pharmaceutical services. The National Health Service in the United Kingdom estimated an expenditure of 2.8 million pounds in 1970 for the treatment of migraine. This was considered an underestimate because an analysis of the cost of treatment at hospital outpatient clinics and of the cost of private expenditure on analgesic drugs was not available (Office of Health Economics, 1972). If we use this figure as a basis for calculation and adjust it for the population of the USA, for inflation and for the higher cost of medical services in the USA (compared to the National Health Service in the United Kingdom) we can estimate that the annual expenditure for migraine in the USA must be well in excess of $100 million.

Loss of working time through migraine must be considered as a further adverse factor for the economy. In the United Kingdom during the year 1968-1969 it was recorded that 295 000 man days and 167 000 woman days were lost through migraine. As these figures include only absences of three consecutive days or more, and exclude all one-day absences which are typical of migraine, they represent a gross underestimate (Office of Health Economics, 1972). If we correct these figures for the USA and assume that the prevalence of migraine is similar in the two countries, we can estimate that migraine accounts for the loss of at least 2 million working days in the United States each year.

These impressive statistical figures take no account of the personal cost of migraine to the patient and to his or her family. The risk of sudden incapacity excludes the migrainous patient from certain occupations. It causes uncertainty and apprehension and often handicaps the patient's lifestyle. Attacks occurring during important events, such as an examination or a job interview, may have serious and long lasting consequences.

Chapter 2

Aetiology

Heredity

The familial occurrence of migraine is beyond doubt. However, it is difficult to obtain reliable data on the frequency of inheritance of migraine, because patients are not often fully informed about the existence and clinical characteristics of headaches in their immediate relatives. Inaccurate information about the family history as well as differences in case material help to explain the wide range in the proportion of 45% to 90% of migrainous patients who have affected relatives quoted in various studies in the literature. When only parents and siblings were considered, Lance and Anthony (1966) obtained a positive family history in 46% of migraineurs compared with only 18% of patients suffering from typical tension headaches. When the family history also included grandparents this figure rose to 55% of 464 patients studied by Selby and Lance (1960). In the large series of cases reported by Friedman *et al.* (1954), the proportion of migraine patients who knew of members of the immediate family similarly affected was 65%. In Bille's (1962) monograph 79.5% of children with severe migraine had parents or siblings suffering from similar headaches; the mother had migraine in 72.6% and the father in 20.5% of these children. Dalsgaard-Nielsen (1965) recorded a familial occurrence of migraine ranging from 75% to 90% of adult migraineurs with various forms of migraine. The family history was on the maternal side in 50% to 70% of these subjects while it occurred in the father in only 16% to 19%. On occasions a family history of migraine can be obtained through three or even five generations. Familial occurrence is much lower in patients with cluster headache, compared to the frequency of a positive family history in classic or common migraine, while it is very much higher in those who suffer from the rare variety of hemiplegic migraine.

There is no definite knowledge nor consensus of opinion on the mode of inheritance. Wolff (1963) assumes that migraine is due to a recessive gene with a penetrance of about 70%, but Refsum (1968) points out that recessive inheritance would result in a higher frequency among siblings than among parents. A high degree of consanguinity has never been demonstrated in the parents of migraine patients. Several authors cited by Refsum (1968) favour dominant inheritance with incomplete penetrance, while Dalsgaard-Nielsen (1965) favours a more complicated inheritance, perhaps resulting from the additive effect of many genes which combine to determine the constitution of the migraine sufferer. A low threshold of pain from vasodilation may be one of the features inherited. While no sex-linkage has been demonstrated in the heredity of migraine, there may be some sex-influence. Refsum (1968) also considers the possibility of multifactorial inheritance, because the expression of dominant genes may be modified by other genes and by environmental factors. The few reported studies of twins have shown only that monozygotic twins are more often concordant than dizygotic twins and have not helped to resolve the conflicting views on the genetic aspects of migraine.

An analysis of many studies available in the literature provides convincing evidence that a predisposition to migraine is transmitted from parent to offspring. As the pathogenesis of migraine involves many factors and is still not fully understood, it remains uncertain what exactly is inherited. Is it some instability of neurovegetative mechanisms, a lack of an enzyme or of a polypeptide concerned with the regulation of arterial constriction and dilatation, or simply a low threshold of pain due to arterial distension? As will be shown later in this chapter, environmental factors contribute to the occurrence of a migraine attack in a susceptible individual. Do some of these patients simply inherit an undue sensitivity to external environmental factors or to physiological changes which do not affect non-migrainous subjects?

In the epidemiological study of Waters (1971), the prevalence of migraine in the families of migrainous subjects did not reach the usually accepted levels of statistical significance. He concludes that heredity is less important than usually supposed. It must be emphasized that in clinical practice the absence of a positive family history cannot be considered as a criterion against a diagnosis of migraine.

Personality Structure

In the absence of controlled studies of personality profiles in migraine sufferers, no specific characteristics of a migraine personality can be laid down. However, some broad generalizations can be made. From observations on a personal series of several thousand patients, it would appear that a patient's personality and psychological make-up play no part in the aetiology of pure classical migraine. They have some significance in the genesis of common migraine and increase in importance in subjects where migraine is combined with tension headaches.

The view that migraine affects mainly intelligent and successful people was disproven by Waters (1971), who found no statistically significant difference in the intelligence scores of about 400 patients, divided into four groups. These groups compared headache-free subjects with those suffering from non-specific headache, unilateral headache, or definite migraine. The fact that intelligent and affluent people are more likely to seek medical advice than the less privileged sections of the community has contributed to the erroneous belief that migraine occurs mainly in the higher social strata and in people who use their brain rather than their muscles.

There are many reports seeking to define a migraine personality which are based on a variety of psychological and psychoanalytical studies and usually rely only on a small number of patients. The consensus is that many migraineurs are compulsive, rigid, perfectionist and ambitious and that a similar proportion is anxious, hyperactive and unable to relax. Some sufferers come from families who have strict norms of behaviour and take pride in achievement. The patient grows up in an environment where attainment is a major goal and anger and aggression must be suppressed. We have, however, no published data on the prevalence of similar personality traits in control groups of people of comparable age, sex and social background who do not suffer from migraine. In a series of 500 patients who came from all social strata and who attended a neurological diagnostic centre an attempt was made to assess the personality of migraine sufferers from questions about their attitudes to stress, anxiety over minor matters and obsessional behaviour patterns (Selby and Lance, 1960). It was found that 23% of these patients exhibited obsessional traits; they were tidy, meticulous, houseproud and in the habit of double checking their actions.

An example of such behaviour was provided by a woman who, while confined to bed in a darkened room with an intolerably severe headache was forced to get up repeatedly and straighten the displaced folds of her curtains.

A similar proportion of this group (22%) admitted that they were unable to relax, restless and overactive, but with only minor psychosomatic symptoms of nervous tension. A further 13% of this series of patients — and these included some who had both migraine and tension headaches — had more overt manifestations of an anxiety state, including insomnia, nervous dyspepsia and a digital tremor, in addition to headache. One-third of these people also suffered from episodic depression unrelated to the timing of headache. Less than one-half (42%) of these 500 patients considered themselves calm, relaxed, not unduly ambitious and without obsessional character traits. It is probable that the proportion of "normal" people would have been smaller if the inquiry into their personality had been more thorough and had relied on scores derived from one of the commonly used personality inventories.

In the absence of hard statistical data we can only propose a theory that the obsessional, tense and hyperactive personality traits presumed to prevail in migraineurs combine with their heredity to lay a fertile "soil" in which the "seeds" or triggers of certain environmental circumstances suffice to bring on an attack of migraine. This theory fits into the fundamental concept that the aetiology of migraine is multifactorial.

Environmental Factors

The extensive literature on migraine refers to an almost inexhaustible list of events and stimuli in the external environment and to changes in the internal physiological milieu which can bring on an attack of migraine. As some of these factors are specific for the individual patient, their elucidation may contribute to more effective treatment. It is neither possible, nor of great importance for the treatment of our patients, to establish statistically valid figures for the relative incidence of each of these triggers. The physician who treats a large number of migraine patients soon realizes that what hurts one may not affect another. The following description of common events in both the external and internal environment which can contribute to a vascular headache may be useful when obtaining the patient's history. Exposure to some, but by no means all, of these "triggers" can be avoided and so achieve a reduction in the frequency of attacks.

External Environment

1. *Climate.* The frequency of migraine attacks often increases in humid and hot weather; it is difficult to decide if this is the direct result of the adverse climate or secondary to fatigue and loss of working efficiency. A few patients

claim that an electric storm invariably precipitates a headache. Westerly winds, particularly in Switzerland and the adjoining provinces of Austria, are said to evoke a significant increase in the occurrence of migraine in the local population. Heyck (1958) elicited a history of a strong relationship between weather and migraine in 45% of 129 patients, while only 16% of Barolin's (1969) patients considered their attacks influenced by climatic changes.

2. *Bright light.* Although no information is available which compares migraine subjects with those who are headache free, sensitivity to glare appears to be one of the prominent characteristics of the migraineur. Of 293 patients specifically questioned 47% regarded glare as an important factor contributing to their migraine attacks (Selby and Lance, 1960). Therefore some patients wear sunglasses most of the time — even in the doctor's surgery. Many have learned to avoid strong light, particularly that reflected from water or snow. A smaller number of migraine subjects report that the flickering light from a movie or television screen will evoke a severe headache either immediately or the next morning. Children often develop vascular headache after attending a movie matinee; the excitement and noise combine with the flickering screen to produce the attack. Surprisingly, the adverse influence of stroboscopic lights at discos and dance halls is only very rarely reported. As only very few people complain of migraine after photic stimulation during the recording of an electroencephalogram, it is possible that the duration of exposure to a strong flickering light is of importance in bringing on headache. In some persons subject to classical migraine, the photic trigger may evoke shimmering scotomata followed by severe headache within 15 to 30 minutes after exposure. The physiological changes relating this sensitivity to bright and shimmering light with the vascular mechanisms of migraine have not yet been elucidated.

3. *Food.* A wide variety of foods can lead to an attack of migraine in individual patients. Chocolate, cheese, fried and fatty foods, oranges, tomatoes and onions are most frequently implicated. Monosodium glutamate, which is usually added to Chinese food, causes headache which is not strictly migrainous and often affects persons not previously subject to migraine.

One of my patients kept a record of what he had eaten on the day preceding each of his frequent migraine attacks. He discovered that apples were the culprit. Three years later he thanked me for "curing" his migraine as not a single attack had occurred since he avoided apples.

In a group of 339 migrainous subjects, where the history contained specific information on diet, one-quarter had discovered a recurring relationship between the headache and prior ingestion of certain foods (Selby and Lance, 1960).

Tyramine is a constituent of many foods which appears to contribute to migraine headache. In a double blind trial of tyramine and lactose, tyramine was convincingly shown to be a migraine precipitant (Smith, Kellow and Hanington, 1970). Tyramine is a vasoactive monoamine, which is deaminated by the monoamine oxidase (MAO) group of enzymes. A controlled study of the metabolism of tyramine in 13 patients with dietary migraine suggested the possibility that they have a deficiency of a conjugating enzyme required for the metabolism of tyramine. Chocolate, however, contains little or no tyramine. Another vasoactive amine, beta phenylethylamine, was identified in chocolate. Many cheeses and some red wines also contain this compound. Careful experimental work has demonstrated a highly significant decrease in phenylethylamine oxidising ability in persons subject to dietary migraine (Sandler *et al.,* 1974). Tyramine and beta phenylethylamine fall into the same group of vasoactive amines as adrenaline and noradrenaline. Other vasoactive amines will probably be identified in foods responsible for dietary migraine. It is postulated that a deficiency in one of the monoamine oxidase (MAO) enzymes results in changes in the metabolism of vasoactive amines which can cause migraine.

There is some doubt whether the occurrence of a migraine headache after the consumption of certain foods is truly an idiosyncrasy or whether it depends on a conditioned reflex. Some authors attribute no importance to dietary triggers and cite experiments with a small number of subjects where the suspect dietary substance, if concealed in a capsule, produced no more headache than a capsule containing lactose or a similar inert substance. This occurred only when the patients did not know what they were taking (Wolff, 1963, pp 445-446). It is difficult to draw useful conclusions from such conflicting reports. The lay press, particularly the periodicals read by women, often presents a list of foods which are claimed to cause migraine. This motivates some people to strictly avoid all these foods without having first experimented to discover whether any of them contribute to their own headache. It is not difficult for an intelligent person to determine if any particular item of food is repeatedly followed by an attack of headache. It does not matter then whether the mechanism is idiosyncratic or a conditioned reflex — such food should be avoided. Reliable, experimental data have suggested that foods containing tyramine and similar vasoactive amines may be significant in migraine; this cannot be dismissed lightly.

4. *Alcohol.* Many migraineurs are emphatic that even small amounts of alcohol will cause an attack. Some authors attribute this simply to the vasodilator effect of ethanol. If this were true, then migraine should occur after the consumption of any alcoholic beverage — beer, wine, spirits or liqueurs. However, the facts are that a major proportion of migraine patients experiences a headache only after drinking even small quantities of fortified wine, such as port, or red wine. In some patients, only a particular variety of grape will evoke an attack. Furthermore, some people not otherwise prone to migraine will experience headache regularly after drinking red wine. In Australia the sale of red wine has declined severely in recent years, even though the quality of the wines is excellent. Market research has shown that this slump is due to a widespread fear of headache. The vintners have changed to growing white grapes and the industry is now fostering research to determine the ingredients in red wine which may be responsible; tyramine, beta phenylethylamine and histamine are under suspicion. As many thousands of people complain of vascular headache after drinking red wine or fortified wine, it cannot be due to a conditioned reflex; a chemical effect of one of the ingredients on the cranial vessels seems more likely.

5. *Hunger.* Attacks of migraine may occur after missed meals. It is suspected, but not proven, that hypoglycaemia and biochemical and physiological changes secondary to this are the cause of such headaches. On the other hand, headache is not a common feature of episodes of hypoglycaemia in insulin dependent diabetics.

6. *Pharmaceutical preparations.* While certain vasoactive drugs may cause vascular headache in most users, persons with migraine are more susceptible to this effect. If possible, nitrites, used for the treatment of ischaemic heart disease, nicotinic acid, reserpine and histamine should not be prescribed for migrainous subjects.

7. *Stress and relaxation.* Though migraine is not primarily a psychogenic illness, stress and excitement are the most common precipitants not only for a single attack, but also for a temporary increase in frequency and severity of headache. The causal impact of stress gains importance in patients where migraine coexists with psychogenic tension headaches. At the other end of the spectrum, stress contributes little to purely classical migraine and hardly at all to cluster headaches. In a group of 388 patients, where specific inquiry for a relationship between migraine and stress situations was made, 67% had recognized such a relationship (Selby and Lance, 1960). In the same patient population, 45% were assessed as either tense and hyperactive or showing obsessional and overambitious personality traits. A further 13% of these subjects had more overt clinical stigmata of an anxiety state. These figures agree, in general, with other studies reported in the literature. We can now propose the concept that an individual predisposed to migraine by heredity and personality structure will develop headache as a reaction to physical or emotional stress. In the eyes of the family, or of the attending physician, the stress may be trivial, but it has a synergistic effect with other "endogenous" precipitants such as lack of sleep and menstruation. A shopping visit to crowded and noisy stores is a recurrent and potent trigger for many young women. They have to rush in the morning to get the children off to school and the house in order, and the rush continues throughout the day to get back home before the children return from school. The worry of preparing a dinner party, the apprehension surrounding examinations or the publication of their results are other common examples from everyday life which bring on a migraine headache. It is not unusual for children with migraine to suffer an attack before a party — here a pleasant anticipation rather than worry is a sufficient stimulus. Many patients can cope better with more severe and sustained environmental stress, such as illness in the family or an economic setback. In some of them the attack of migraine will occur only after the adverse circumstances have been resolved.

A moderate proportion of the migraine population experiences headache mainly during periods of relaxation. The term "weeekend headache" has been used to describe the recurrent sufferings of these unfortunate people. They will predictably have an attack almost every Saturday or Sunday, particularly if the preceding week was stressful and not all the set goals and ambitions could be achieved. Others report migraine (at times, of exeeptional severity) on the first day of every vacation. A period of intense activity and lack of sleep, rushing to get work and projects completed in time — and to perfection — before the holiday, contribute to the changes in autonomic function and cranial vascular tone which find their clinical expression in an attack of migraine. The often quoted assumption that the cranial vasculature also relaxes during periods of mental and physical relaxation is surely an oversimplification of a large number of complex physiological events which involve mainly the autonomic nervous system.

Internal Environment

This term is used to describe sustained, recurrent or cyclic physiological events which may be associated with migraine, but which cannot always be manipulated by the patient.

1. *Menstruation.* While it is clear that the occurrence of migraine in many

women is closely linked to the menstrual cycle, the hormonal factors and changes in fluid balance which may be responsible for this association are still a subject of controversy. Some 62% of 196 women reported a temporal relationship between attacks of migraine and menstruation or ovulation (Selby and Lance, 1960). The headache may occur during the premenstrual week, or during or immediately after the menses. It is not often a fixed or predictable relationship to specific phases of the cycle: one month, the headache occurs during the premenstrual days; the next month, it is delayed until the end of the flow. In a small proportion of women, migraine occurs exclusively at the time of the menses. In these patients, daily measurements of the plasma concentrations of progesterone and oestradiol indicated that migraine is precipitated by the rapid lowering of plasma oestradiol or one of its metabolites in the premenstrual phase. An injection of oestradiol valerate delayed the onset of migraine in these women for three to nine days (Somerville, 1972a).

However, other contributions to the vast literature on "hormonal migraine" have postulated raised levels of oestrogen and a sudden fall of circulating progestogens at the time of headache. Therapeutic successes were claimed for the administration of various hormone preparations: oestrogens; progestogens; gonadotrophins; and even androgens. The majority of therapeutic trials were uncontrolled and the same degree of success was often not achieved by other investigators. At present no specific hormone preparation can be recommended for the prevention of menstrual migraine.

During pregnancy migraine tends to improve and may even cease. In a study of 200 pregnant women, 31 had suffered from migraine before conception had taken place. In 24 of these (77%) the headaches improved (Somerville, 1972a). Other authors have reported that from 50% to 87% of migrainous women enjoy a respite from headache while they are pregnant. On the other hand, a small proportion of previously non-migrainous women may experience the first attack of migraine during pregnancy. This happened to only 5% of the subjects studied by Somerville (1972b). The reason for this temporary improvement in migraine during pregnancy is not clear. The assumption that raised levels of progesterone may inhibit vasomotor responses of cranial arteries is not supported by studies which show that progesterone values are no different in those subjects who improve from those subjects who continue to have migraine while pregnant.

Vascular headaches may begin at the time of the menarche and frequently, but by no means invariably, improve or even disappear at the menopause. Therefore attention was focused on the importance of changes in hormone levels for the pathogenesis of menstrual migraine, while other physiological events or changes in emotional tone during certain phases of the menstrual cycle were relatively neglected. One of these is fluid retention, which sometimes occurs just before and during an attack of migraine; a brisk diuresis may then occur as the headache subsides. During the premenstrual phase there is weight gain and, at times, oedema indicative of fluid retention. However, the deliberate induction of water retention does not regularly provoke an attack of migraine, nor does its relief invariably curtail it. Oestradiol may cause fluid retention indirectly through changes in water and electrolyte balance mediated by the hypothalamic-posterior pituitary axis, which is also involved in other facets of autonomic regulation. Therefore, it would appear that water retention and menstrual migraine have a common origin rather than a cause and effect relationship (Greene, 1962).

The premenstrual syndrome includes changes in emotional tone and behaviour, including irritability and depression. These can create problems in the patient's relationship with her family or workmates, feelings of remorse or guilt, and so may contribute to the precipitation of a migraine attack in a predisposed individual. This great variety of potential trigger factors helps to explain why the majority of women do not have headaches predictably during the same phase of the cycle and may remain free of migraine in some cycles. In spite of the obvious deficiencies in our knowledge of the mechanisms involved in the causation of vascular headaches associated with menstruation, there are some women who request hysterectomy in the vain hope that it will "cure" their migraine. They have heard that migraine often ceases after the menopause and seem convinced that uterine bleeding is an essential cause of their suffering. Unfortunately some gynaecologists accede to their request, but most of these women later return to their physicians complaining of migraine of the same frequency and severity, though no longer linked to a menstrual flow. In many the condition is worse because of complex and partly subconscious psychological mechanisms consequent on the loss of the uterus.

Strong and dogmatic opinions are often expressed that migraine is caused, or at least aggravated, by oral contraceptives. The daily papers and periodical magazines, always in pursuit of sensational news, have given this subject more publicity than the scientific literature. It is true that some women, while they are taking ovulation inhibitors, experience vascular headaches for the first time and that in some the frequency or severity of pre-existing migraine increases. In others, however, the same contraceptive tablets cause a significant improvement in migraine. Neither the oestrogen nor the progesterone component of these preparations was convincingly shown to have a predominant effect on the occurrence or absence of headache. Many women have tried a multitude of different pills, containing various doses and combinations of oestrogens and progestogens, without achieving any change in the pattern of their headache. These observations are consistent with the lack of evidence for any specific hormonal changes in the pathogenesis of menstrual migraine. In clinical practice, dogmatic preconceived ideas should be avoided; only clinical trial will establish if an individual woman's migraine is worse or better while she is taking oral contraceptive tablets.

2. *Physical or mental exhaustion.* Some patients state that their attacks of migraine are temporally related to excessive fatigue, which can result either from prolonged physical exertion or mental and intellectual performance. This is the opposite to the more common occurrence of migraine during times of relaxation. Exhaustion is hardly ever the sole trigger for every attack such a person suffers. It provides only a further example of the multiplicity of events which, alone or in combination with other triggers, can push susceptible individuals beyond the brink of their relatively low limits of tolerance and result in the vascular and autonomic changes of common migraine.

In children, migraine occurs frequently in the afternoon after playing games, particularly on hot and glary days. The physical exertion, resulting in cutaneous vasodilation, exposure to bright light, and the excitement of the game combine to produce the headache, which usually lasts only an hour or two.

3. *Sleep.* Weekend or vacation migraine frequently occurs when the patient sleeps in. This was reported by 44 of 138 migrainous patients studied by Heyck (1958). The histories provided by patients indicate that headache appears after rising late in the morning, and not after an equal duration of sleep if the patient

retires to bed early. Experimental work has shown that the onset of migraine during sleep or on waking occurs mainly during or immediately after a rapid eye movement (REM) phase of sleep. This has not yet been explained satisfactorily. This specific trigger for weekend headaches should always be ascertained from the history, because the patient can easily avoid attacks by getting up as early on weekends as on working days.

4. *Hypertension.* There are conflicting reports on the incidence and significance of hypertension in migraine. Moser *et al.* (1962) found that only 20.5% of their 556 patients with hypertension and headache had vascular headaches of the migraine type. As their paper is concerned only with people who suffered from both hypertension and headache, this fairly small proportion of migraine implies that the prevalence of migraine in the general hypertensive population is not significantly different from that in normotensive people. Blood pressure readings exceeded 20.0kPa (150mm Hg) systolic and 13.3kPa (100mm Hg) diastolic in only 13% of the 500 patients with migraine studied by Selby and Lance (1960). Although the ages of the hypertensive patients are not stated, the frequency of hypertension in the non-migrainous population is not significantly different. Walker (1959), in disagreement with most other authors, found a remarkably high incidence of 52% of migraine in his series of hypertensive patients. The blood pressure of migrainous subjects over the age of 50 years was higher than in controls. He concluded from this that migraineurs are more likely to develop hypertension in later life than the general population.

There is some consensus of opinion that the onset of hypertension may increase the frequency and severity of migraine headache. The more forceful thrust of the increased arterial pulse pressure is now added to the deficient vasomotor tone and increased pain sensitivity of extracranial arteries. The headache responds to vasoconstrictor drugs, such as ergotamines, even though they cause a temporary rise in blood pressure. Treatment of the hypertension usually reduces the frequency and severity of headache to their pre-hypertensive levels.

The diverse factors, both in the "external" environment and in the "internal" physiological milieu are not linked by a common denominator. Some of them have an influence on cranial vascular tone by various mechanisms, which may be physical (barometric and temperature changes), hormonal, or biochemical (induced by vasoactive components of certain foods). Others have no apparent direct action on the cranial vasculature, but may affect autonomic regulation either through the hypothalamus or through more peripheral parts of the autonomic nervous system. The fundamental concept is that persons subject to common migraine differ from the much larger non-migrainous population in their susceptibility to these extraneous and endogenous stimuli. This is a qualitative and not a quantitative difference.

Autonomic Instability

There is good clinical evidence that the disturbance of autonomic regulation in the migraine syndrome extends beyond its impact on intracranial and extracranial vessels. A considerable proportion of adult migraineurs have a past history of "cyclic vomiting" or of the related "recurrent syndrome" during childhood. The symptoms consist either of recurrent episodes of unprovoked and often severe vomiting, or of repeated attacks of abdominal pain, nausea, pallor and fever. It is not surprising that acute appendicitis is suspected during the initial attacks and that the true diagnosis becomes obvious only when the symptoms subside spontaneously, to recur later in an episodic fashion and at irregular intervals. Headache may be relatively inconspicuous during the attacks in early childhood. Toddlers with "cyclic vomiting" may develop repetitive attacks of abdominal pain at the age of three or four years, and progress to episodes of headache, sometimes alternating with abdominal pain, when they reach the age of seven to ten.

Almost one-third of 198 patients with vascular headache recalled frequently recurring and severe bilious attacks during childhood, though the inquiry extended beyond the strict definition of "cyclic vomiting". In a larger proportion (59%) of a further 139 migrainous patients a history of some bilious attacks or of severe motion sickness during childhood and adolescence was obtained (Selby and Lance, 1960). An epidemiological study by Waters (1972) found that a past history of bilious attacks in both sexes and of travel sickness in males (but not females) was significantly more common in the migrainous group than in the rest of the population.

Analysis of the case histories of migraine patients reveals that a major proportion shows various other clinical manifestations of instability of the autonomic nervous system. These include dizziness on standing up, syncopal episodes brought on by emotional or physical determinants, and considerable fluctuations in blood pressure levels. Dysmenorrhoea appears to be prevalent in migrainous women. Cold hands and feet, sometimes accompanied by pallor or cyanosis, demonstrate the excessive reactivity of peripheral vascular tone. Experimental work has suggested that the hands of migrainous subjects show a poor vasodilator response to heat; it is not certain whether this is due to an abnormal responsiveness of peripheral vessels, or to some defect in the central regulating mechanism of autonomic control. Nausea and vomiting, changes in fluid and electrolyte balance, and oliguria or polyuria, which may be associated with the attacks of migraine headache, are further examples of autonomic dysfunction. With the exception of bilious attacks in childhood, I am not aware of any epidemiological studies which compare the incidence of autonomic instability in migraine patients with the general population. Further attention to this relatively neglected aspect of the disease could produce helpful clues towards a solution of the enigma of migraine.

Trauma

While the economic stresses and emotional reactions consequent upon severe head injuries may increase the frequency and severity of attacks in migraine subjects, the appearance of migraine for the first time after severe cranial trauma is unusual. An exception to this is the onset of a localized vascular headache shortly after traumatic contusion of an extracranial artery. The trauma is usually of minor degree and the vessels may be damaged by laceration of the overlying scalp or by a blunt injury. It is assumed that damage to the periarterial sympathetic plexus can cause an abnormality in the binding of noradrenaline to the adventitia of these arteries, which renders them more susceptible to painful dilatation. Holland (1976) described three such cases, where the pain was localized to the region of the injured artery and its branches; one of these had features consistent with cluster headache, though the attacks occurred every night for over a year. None of the patients responded adequately to conventional drug treatment for migraine, but in all three cases surgical ligation of the involved artery achieved dramatic and complete relief. Cases of classical migraine precipitated by head trauma and following the same pattern in later recurring attacks have also been reported (Matthews, 1972). Here the causal mechanisms are more difficult to explain and the pathogenetic relationship must extend well beyond injury to a branch of the superficial temporal artery.

Migraine and Epilepsy

Opinions concerning the relationship between migraine and epilepsy are still conflicting. Both are paroxysmal disorders which may involve different parts of the brain. Classical migraine shows some clinical similarities to partial epilepsy in that the angiospastic focal cerebral symptoms may occur without ensuing headache, just as an epileptic aura need not be followed by impairment of consciousness. In isolated cases a similar sensory aura may precede either a seizure or a migraine headache. However, when we compare the aetiological and clinical features of the many forms of epilepsy with the characteristics of migraine and its variants, it becomes apparent that differences far outweigh similarities.

As both migraine and epilepsy are not uncommon conditions, their association in the same individual or same family may be explained by chance. Attempts to resolve this question by statistical methods are handicapped by difficulties in a precise diagnostic assessment of both diseases, when often only a vague or indefinite history is available. In a comparison of 1830 cases of migraine with 548 patients suffering from tension headaches, Basser (1969) found an incidence of epilepsy of 5.9% in the migraine group, compared with only 1.1% in the tension headache group. It will be noted that the frequency of epilepsy even in the patients suffering from tension headaches was about double the 0.6% usually quoted for the general population. In our series of 348 patients suffering from migraine and allied vascular headache, 38 (11%) gave a history of childhood convulsions, or of epilepsy not directly associated with migraine attacks (Selby and Lance, 1960). The high incidence of "epilepsy" in this group is largely due to the inclusion of childhood convulsions. In the same study, 15% of 439 patients were found to have a family history of epilepsy in either parents or siblings. In contrast with these figures, which appear to favour a relationship between migraine and epilepsy, Lance and Anthony (1966) found that only 1.6% of 500 migrainous patients had a personal history of epilepsy compared with 2% of 100 patients with psychogenic muscle contraction headache, who attended the same clinic. No significant difference in the family history of epilepsy was found in these two groups of patients. Friedman (1968) also found no statistical evidence in his large series of patients that epilepsy and migraine are related.

The different views and data quoted above serve to emphasize the need for further study. Whitty (1972) approached the problem by considering nosographic similarities, the genetic background, and electroencephalographic (EEG) findings. While admitting that none of these three lines of inquiry provides unequivocal answers, they favour more than a chance association. He considers that migraine and seizures may be linked by a common constitutional factor.

The concept of "dysrhythmic migraine" was proposed by Weil (1952) to describe migrainous patients where the EEG showed abnormalities (dysrhythmias) similar to those seen in some forms of epilepsy. Several later studies have shown that from 20% to 43% of migraine subjects have "dysrhythmic" EEGs irrespective of the association of focal cerebral disturbances with the headache. However, in the majority of cases the EEG patterns are not specifically epileptic; they consist mainly of excessive slow activity, which may be persistent or episodic and shows a focal emphasis in only a modest proportion of cases. It was fashionable to treat "dysrhythmic migraine" with anticonvulsant drugs, but the results were never spectacular. On the contrary, the failure of anticonvulsant drugs in the prevention of migraine may be used as evidence against a link between migraine and epilepsy.

Focal cerebral ischaemia can result from severe intracranial angiospasm during an attack of classical or complicated migraine. Such an area of ischaemia may later become an epileptogenic focus and explain the appearance of partial or generalized seizures in a patient with a preceding history of migraine. It is surprising that this sequence of events is relatively uncommon.

In clinical practice the association between migraine and seizures, particularly if the latter are partial (focal), should always arouse the suspicion of a cortical arteriovenous malformation (angioma). However, loss of consciousness may occur also from other causes at the height of an attack of severe migraine. In most of these cases, convulsive movements, tongue biting and sphincter relaxation do not occur. The duration of coma is usually brief and it is not easy to distinguish between migraine-syncope and migraine-epilepsy. Loss of consciousness is a feature of the relatively rare condition of "basilar" migraine, but it may also be caused by a more diffuse constriction of intracranial vessels, combined with fluid and electrolyte changes due to vomiting during a severe attack of common or classical migraine.

It is reasonable to assume that a person predisposed to epilepsy, genetically or otherwise, is more prone to have a seizure in association with a migraine attack. While some would interpret this as a common genetic constitution, it does not really lend strength to the arguments in favour of a link between migraine and epilepsy.

Relationship of Migraine with Allergic Disorders

An allergic background to migraine was favoured in the literature before 1960. The authors of most papers were specifically interested in allergic diseases and this introduced a bias in the case material they studied and reported. Often no clear distinction was drawn between food and inhalant allergens. Diagnostic difficulties and differences in the definition of migraine contributed further to the discrepancies in the findings and conclusions. Specific inquiry for a past history of common allergic diseases, including asthma, vasomotor rhinitis, urticaria and eczema, elicited a positive response from 35% of 311 patients; in the same study 38% of 330 patients had a positive family history (including both parents and siblings) of such allergic disorders (Selby and Lance, 1960). These figures are considerably higher than the incidence of similar allergic manifestations in the community, which is estimated to lie between 5% and 10%. The severity and persistence of allergic diseases in this group of migrainous subjects is not stated, but they probably included patients who mentioned only isolated attacks of allergic rhinitis or urticaria during childhood. This would help to explain why later studies by other authors found a much lower frequency of similar allergic illness. For example, Lance and Anthony (1966) found no significant difference in the personal or family histories of allergic illness in 500 migrainous subjects compared with 100 patients suffering from muscle contraction headache. Also we must recognize that persons with a known allergic diathesis may have quite unrelated vascular headaches. On rare occasions, however, an attack of migraine can occur at the same time as an allergic illness. Kallós and Kallós-Deffner (1955) described 28 of a group of 185 migraine patients with associated allergic diseases, where an attack of migraine was repeatedly precipitated by exposure to a specific allergen and occurred simultaneously with allergic rhinitis, asthma or angioneurotic oedema.

The occurrence of migraine after the ingestion of foods containing vasoactive amines, such as tyramine, cannot be considered as an argument in favour of a relationship between migraine and allergy. Inhalant allergens, such as pollens, will cause migraine only in isolated instances. This happened to one of my patients:

A man with a past history of allergic rhinitis and a family history of allergy experienced daily attacks of typical migraine only in July of each year over a period of 11 years. The attacks then ceased for six years while he was living in other cities. They recurred when he returned to his original home, which was close to wattle trees. The seasonal occurrence of his migraine was related to wattle blossoms and he was found to be intensely allergic to them. However, the same patient developed attacks of migraine unrelated to this allergen some years later.

The importance of histamine, 5-hydroxytryptamine (serotonin) and of a polypeptide, bradykinin, in the pathogenesis of changes in vascular calibre in migraine was established by many experimental studies in recent years. The fact that the same substances are known to appear as a result of antigen-antibody interaction cannot be accepted as a valid argument in favour of a causal relationship between migraine and allergy.

The observations cited above do not provide convincing clinical or laboratory evidence for the importance of "allergic" factors in the aetiology or pathogenesis of common or classical migraine. The same may not apply to cluster headache, which has both clinical and biochemical differences from other varieties of migraine. As histamine and not serotonin was shown to be involved in the pathogenesis of cluster headache, Anthony (1972b) has proposed the hypothesis that it may be an "allergic" disorder.

The assessment of a patient with migraine should include inquiry for the coexistence of any of the common allergic diseases. Only in the rare cases where the history suggests a relationship between inhalant antigens and the occurrence of a migraine attack may the performance of appropriate skin tests and desensitization injections prove to be rewarding.

From the multitude of factors which are widely recognized as potentially contributing to migraine we can now construct a concept for its pathogenesis. This applies mainly to common migraine, but may play a part in classical migraine and in some other variants of the syndrome (Fig. 1).

A predisposition to migraine is determined partly by heredity and partly by the patient's personality and constitution. This predisposition includes an un-

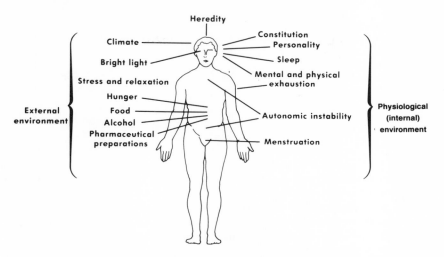

Fig. 1. Some of the factors in the patient's external and internal environment which can bring on a migraine attack.

stable neurovegetative (autonomic) system which can manifest itself already in early childhood. The susceptibility to migraine persists throughout patients' lives, constantly exposing them to the risks of an attack — the jug is nearly full but will overflow if only a few more drops are added. Additional "triggers" are needed to produce the autonomic and vascular changes, which find their clinical expression in headache and in the other symptoms of a migraine attack. These "triggers" may be either physiological events, such as menstruation or anomalies in the pattern and duration of rapid eye movement (REM) sleep, or they may come from the external environment, particularly stress situations and, less often, from exposure to bright light or the consumption of certain foods and beverages. Migraineurs are rarely susceptible only to a single specific trigger for their attacks. Most of them will respond to a variety of external and physiological events. A combination of several external and internal determinants will greatly increase the chances of an attack and will also contribute to a temporary increase in frequency, but not severity. There are other reasons why the pain in some attacks is more severe than in others; these include the degree of cranial vascular distension, with its concomitant oedema and the individual's tolerance or intolerance to pain. The patient's constitution and personality structure will also determine which of the protean internal and external events are the most potent in evoking attacks.

Fundamentally, an attack of migraine is the product of patients' abnormal susceptibility and of their aberrant reactions to internal and external stimuli.

Chapter 3

Pathogenesis

Pathophysiology

It is generally accepted from experimental and clinical evidence that migraine is associated with an abnormal reactivity of blood vessels both in the brain and in the scalp. However, we must recognize that changes in the calibre of intracranial and extracranial vessels cannot be the primary or sole cause of either the focal neurological symptoms or of the headache of a migraine attack.

The experimental work and clinical observations of Wolff and his colleagues over a period of 25 years are presented in *Headache and Other Head Pain* (Wolff, 1963). He clearly established that cranial vessels constrict during the pre-headache phase, but distend at the time of the headache. Oedema of the extra-cranial arterial wall, which then becomes rigid, was shown to occur in the late headache phase and for some time afterwards. These concepts appeared to provide a satisfactory explanation of events which occur during various stages of a migraine attack. However, they left many questions unanswered which became the focus of further study in recent years.

Changes in Intracranial Vessels

The retinal and cerebral symptoms which may occur before or during a migraine headache are traditionally attributed to constriction of intracranial vessels and to the resultant focal cerebral ischaemia. Retinal arterial constriction was observed in a few instances where a patient's optic fundus could be examined during a migrainous scotoma. There are also reports of isolated cases where visual scotomata occurred during cerebral angiography — in some the films showed reduced filling of the branches of the internal carotid artery when the patient experienced visual or focal neurological disturbances, while cerebral perfusion was normal during the headache phase. The validity of these angiographic observations has been questioned on the grounds that the injection of the contrast medium itself may have precipitated the changes in vascular calibre.

Other studies, using radioactive xenon either by inhalation or intra-carotid injection (O'Brien, 1970; Skinhøj, 1970) have shown a significant reduction in regional cortical flow during the prodromal phase and an increase in perfusion at the height of the headache. However, in one of these studies the reduction in cerebral blood flow affected both hemispheres equally and did not correlate with the clinical localization of the migraine aura.

Transient focal electroencephalographic abnormalities were observed from the occipital lobes and other regions of the brain during migrainous visual field defects and disturbances of speech, sensation or movement in the premonitory phase of a migraine attack. It is generally held that these are the result of isch-aemia caused by intracranial angiospasm.

There may be secondary changes contributing to this tissue ischaemia such as swelling of the vascular endothelium and loss of intravascular fluid through increased permeability of vessel walls. These tend to resolve within 20 to 30 minutes, a timespan corresponding with the average duration of most migraine prodromata. Another theory, based mainly on the clinical characteristics of some migrainous scotomata, postulates a peak of excitation followed by a wave of cortical depression. Such a mechanism could apply only to the small number of patients who experience an advancing crescent of scintillating light (stimulation) followed by loss of vision (inhibition). The rate of progress of these visual phe-nomena in isolated, but well documented, cases is similar to the "spreading depression" described by Leão (1944) in animal brains under conditions which are not strictly comparable to the events which occur in the majority of migraine subjects.

Constriction of intracranial vessels is always transient and is followed by dilation of the same vessels. The *intracranial* arterial distension contributes little, if at all, to the headache phase of a migraine attack. In contrast to pain induced by the injection of histamine, migraine headache is not relieved by raising the cerebrospinal fluid (CSF) pressure up to 1000mm of water, which would com-press and "cushion" the distended intracranial vessels.

The influence of the sympathetic nervous system on the calibre of intra-cranial arteries is weak and insignificant. Vasoactive amines are now thought to be more important than primarily neurogenic stimuli in controlling vascular tone. These vasoactive amines appear to have more effect on the microcirculation, which consists of small arterioles, capillaries and venules, than on large and medium sized vessels. An attractive theory, first proposed by Heyck (1956), sug-gests that tissue ischaemia can result from a temporary shunt which allows blood to flow more directly from feeding arteries into draining veins. The arteriovenous oxygen difference was significantly reduced during an attack of migraine with focal cerebral symptoms. The microcirculation may be constricted while the larger feeding arteries are dilated; this contributes to the shunt mechanism as well as to the more direct tissue ischaemia in the area of capillary constriction.

In summary, data derived from a variety of experimental methods have shown that cerebral blood flow decreases temporarily during the prodromal phase of a migraine attack. This decrease usually affects both hemispheres, but may be relatively greater in the area which correlates with the symptoms experienced by the patient. The causes for these differences in regional perfusion have not been discovered. Cerebral blood flow increases again during the headache phase and it is thought that vasoconstriction and vasodilation may occur simultane-ously in different areas of the brain (Lance, 1972a). The focal or diffuse changes in cerebral perfusion may well be influenced more by the microcirculation than by the calibre of larger vessels. The significance of changes in the vascular wall and in the chemical constitution of the blood within these vessels is now re-ceiving increasing attention and will be discussed later.

Changes in Extracranial Vessels

The work of Wolff and his collaborators (1963) suggested that the pain of migraine was caused by dilation of the arteries of the scalp; the superficial temporal artery and its branches are more often involved than other branches of the external carotid tree. Many patients and their doctors have observed tenderness, swelling and increased pulsation of these scalp vessels. This tenderness may persist after the swelling has subsided and the calibre of the artery has returned to normal. Direct pressure on the distended arteries, or compression of the carotid in the neck, will temporarily diminish the intensity of the pain. The skin on the affected side may be flushed or pale and the small conjunctival vessels are usually dilated.

Clinical and experimental observations (Wolff, 1963) have demonstrated that the "tone" of the distended extracranial arterial wall is reduced. This permits an increased amplitude of pulsation of scalp arteries, which correlates with the severity of headache. An injection of ergotamine restores extracranial arterial tone, reduces the amplitude of pulsation and relieves the headache (Fig. 2). During the prodromal phase of a migraine attack, such as a visual scotoma, the amplitude of pulsation of the superficial temporal artery is lower than during a headache-free period; it then increases greatly on the affected side during the headache phase. The abnormally increased perfusion of scalp vessels was confirmed by experimental tissue clearance studies with radioactive sodium; these showed an increased blood flow in the frontotemporal scalp, but not in the forearm during a migraine headache. Similar to intracranial perfusion, measured by xenon, the increased scalp flow is also bilateral, but relatively greater on the side of hemicrania.

The sympathetic nervous system has much less control of arteries of the scalp than of the vasculature of the limbs. It is involved mainly in vasodilator reflexes. Sympathectomy or chemical blockade of the cervical sympathetic outflow can abolish blushing, but does not increase the amplitude of pulsation of the superficial temporal artery.

If distension and excessive pulsation of scalp vessels were the only cause of the pain in migraine, why does vigorous physical exertion or sunburn of a bald head in a non-migrainous subject fail to produce a similar headache? The exclusive importance of arterial distension in the scalp was challenged also by the observation that a majority of patients are very pale on the side of hemicrania at the peak of a headache. Thermographic studies before and during a migraine headache have shown that the skin temperature becomes lower on the painful side. This is attributed to constriction of arterioles, capillaries and venules, the microcirculation, while the larger arteries are distended. Blood is thus shunted away from the skin by arteriovenous anastomoses which by-pass the constricted capillary bed (Lance and Anthony, 1971). The lower skin temperature on the affected side persists even after the headache is relieved by administration of ergotamine, which constricts the dilated scalp arteries.

We do not know why these fluctuations in extracranial vascular calibre occur only in migrainous subjects, why they are often confined to one half of the cranium or even to a single branch of an extracranial artery, nor do we have any knowledge of the primary mechanisms which precipitate these transient abnormal vascular reactions.

Why does the initial distension of scalp vessels progress to oedema and rigidity of the arterial wall? This sequence of events appears to be specific for migraine and has not been observed in other conditions or in vessels other than those of the scalp. The explanation may be found in cellular or humoral changes which occur in or near the arterial wall in migraine. The experimental evidence

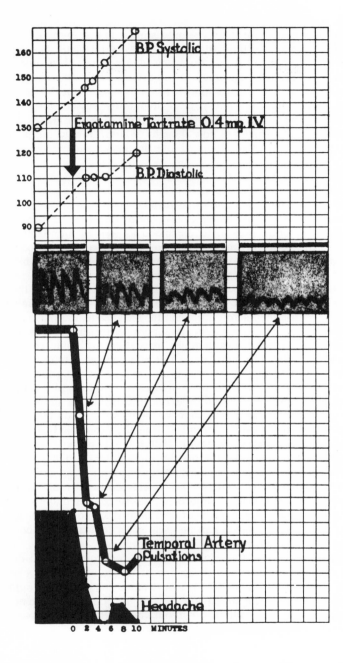

Fig. 2. The amplitude of pulsations of the temporal artery is high when headache is intense. An injection of ergotamine tartrate reduces the amplitude of temporal artery pulsations and relieves headache (reproduced from *Headache and Other Head Pain,* 2nd Edition, 1963, by Harold G. Wolff, with the permission of Oxford University Press).

for a sterile inflammatory reaction in the wall of migrainous scalp arteries was summarized by Wolff (1963). A polypeptide, similar to that found in blister fluid, is present in the periarterial fluid around these vessels during the headache phase. Chapman *et al.* (1960) called this fluid neurokinin. Since then other humoral agents, which are probably adsorbed to the arterial wall, such as serotonin (5-HT) and bradykinin, have been implicated in the causation of the sterile inflammatory reaction of distended and painful migrainous vessels. Both neurokinin and bradykinin were shown to be potent pain provoking substances. These, and other chemical agents which are now thought to contribute to the pathogenesis of migraine headache, will be discussed later in this chapter.

The Platelet Hypothesis

During the last ten years abnormal platelet behaviour in migraine has received considerable attention. As platelets contain almost all the 5-hydroxytryptamine (5-HT, serotonin) present in the blood as well as monoamine oxidase (MAO, an enzyme concerned in the breakdown of vasoactive monoamines) the platelet hypothesis provides a link between some physiological and biochemical events concerned in the pathogenesis of migraine.

Hanington's review of experimental work (1979) has shown that the platelets of migraine sufferers aggregate more readily than those of non-migrainous controls. Platelets release their serotonin when they aggregate and plasma serotonin levels fall during a migraine headache. In support of this hypothesis, Hanington (1979) points out that the catecholamines adrenaline and noradrenaline as well as arachidonic acid and thrombin also affect platelet aggregation. Stress, certain dietary items and hypoglycaemia, which are frequent triggers for an attack of common migraine, are associated with changes in catecholamine output, while hormonal changes influence thrombin levels. In this manner the aggregation of platelets is increased in response to some of the most common migraine precipitants. Aspirin, which is sometimes effective in the prophylaxis of migraine, is a potent inhibitor of platelet aggregation. Hilton (1971) proposes that there may be a *permanent* abnormality of the platelet membrane of migrainous subjects. It seems likely that migrainous platelets accept serotonin less readily or that the receptor sites on the platelet membranes retain serotonin molecules less efficiently than in non-migrainous subjects. It was suggested that the significant difference in the uptake mechanism of serotonin into blood platelets between migrainous and control subjects can be used as an indication of the predisposition of an individual to migraine.

It is not unreasonable to postulate that the prodromal retinal or cerebral symptoms of a migraine attack can be due to the combined effect of platelet aggregation in small vessels and of vasoconstriction following serotonin release. This hypothesis would help to explain the not uncommon occurrence of scotomata and focal cerebral symptoms without ensuing headache in patients with either a past or concurrent history of migraine.

Biochemistry

We have shown earlier that erratic behaviour of the blood vessels of the brain and scalp is fundamental to the pathogenesis of the migraine syndrome.

It was pointed out that the larger vessels react independently from the micro-circulation and that small vessels may be constricted while larger ones dilate. Variations in the calibre of these blood vessels result from changes in the "tone" of their muscular walls. Vascular "tone" is a state of partial contraction of these muscular walls, which is determined partly by neurogenic stimulation and partly by chemical agents. The microcirculation is predominantly under the control of vasoactive chemical agents. These include amines, polypeptides, lipids and hormones.

Vasoactive Amines

The amines which have so far been studied for their role in migraine are some catecholamines, 5-hydroxytryptamine (5-HT, serotonin), histamine and ty-ramine.

1. *Catecholamines (noradrenaline and adrenaline).* Although the infusion of noradrenaline causes constriction of extracranial vessels, there is as yet no clinical or experimental evidence to implicate catecholamines in the pathogenesis of mi-graine. Blood levels of noradrenaline and adrenaline do not vary significantly before, during or after an attack of migraine headache (Anthony, 1972a).

2. *Serotonin (5-HT).* This amine is formed and stored in the gut and enters the circulation via the portal system. It is found almost entirely in platelets, which appear to absorb it from the plasma and can discharge it back into the plasma. Serotonin constricts large arteries and veins and dilates arterioles and capillaries. It is metabolized to 5-hydroxy-indoleacetic acid (5-HIAA) which is excreted in the urine. Sicuteri *et al.* (1961) first reported that the urinary excre-tion of 5-HIAA rises during attacks of migraine. Plasma serotonin levels were found to fall significantly during migraine headache in 80% of patients tested (Curran, Hinterberger and Lance, 1965). The fall of plasma serotonin levels ranges from 9% to 80%, with a mean of 20%. This appears to be specific for migraine headache and does not occur during the severe headache caused by pneumoen-cephalography or during the performance of other stressful procedures. It is highly significant that plasma serotonin levels do not fall during cluster headache.

The intramuscular injection of reserpine lowers plasma serotonin levels and evokes a typical migraine headache in most, but not all, migraine subjects. In a smaller proportion of patients, intravenous serotonin was found to alleviate both spontaneous and reserpine-induced migraine.

If plasma collected during a migraine headache is incubated with platelets collected during a headache-free period, serotonin is released. Therefore, the presence of a serotonin-releasing factor in the plasma during a migraine headache has been postulated. The nature of this factor is as yet undetermined, though a large variety of substances of low molecular weight, including monoamines, poly-peptides, prostaglandins and plasma free fatty acids, are receiving experimental attention.

Serotonin injected into the human common carotid artery causes strong con-striction of extracranial arteries, but makes little difference to the calibre of cere-bral arteries. If serotonin is applied directly to the exposed cerebral cortex the large cerebral arteries will constrict. In contrast, arterioles and capillaries in most parts of the body, including the scalp, are usually dilated by serotonin, but this effect is thought to depend on the degree of pre-existing vascular tone. In the perfused rabbit auricular artery, serotonin was found to enhance the vasoconstrictor effect of sympathetic nerve stimulation as well as of adrenaline, noradrenaline, angiotensin and histamine (de la Lande *et al.*, 1966). However, it is well known that the effect of serotonin on vascular calibre differs in various animal species and it is not certain if this reaction in the rabbit is also applicable to man.

We have sound experimental evidence that plasma serotonin levels fall during a migraine headache. Why then are anti-serotonin drugs such as methysergide and pizotifen often effective in the prophylaxis of migraine? It was suggested that methysergide may occupy receptor sites on the arterial wall and so block the vascular responses to fluctuations in levels of serotonin in the plasma. Another theory proposes that methysergide may have a direct constrictor effect on the carotid tree.

Although serotonin still holds pride of place among all the chemical agents investigated in the pathogenesis of migraine, many questions about its mode of action remain unanswered. In a critical appraisal of the serotonin theory, Somerville (1976) points out that platelets all over the body are losing serotonin equally. Why then do only the vessels of the scalp and brain respond to diminished serotonin in such an abnormal manner? Although there appear to be no anatomical or histochemical differences between cranial arteries and those elsewhere in the body, a varying sensitivity of arteries to both serotonin and methysergide in different sites of the arterial tree has been demonstrated. The mechanisms contributing to such regional variations in arterial "sensitivity" should be the subject of further study, because they would help to explain both the hemicranial situation of many migraine attacks as well as the focal features of migraine prodromata.

3. *Histamine.* Histamine is generally regarded as a vasodilator substance. Headache produced by the injection of histamine is due mainly to distension of intracranial vessels. It occurs after and not during maximal vascular dilation, it is bilateral and not analogous to migraine headache. The mean blood levels of histamine do not rise significantly before, during or after a migraine headache (Anthony, 1972a). We may conclude that histamine plays no part in the pathogenesis of common or classic migraine. However, it appears to be of major importance in cluster headache where significantly raised levels of whole blood histamine have been recorded during attacks (Anthony and Lance, 1971).

Histamine induces a generalized vascular dilation which includes the capillary beds. The release of histamine also causes the concurrent acceleration of its formation in various tissues where the newly formed histamine then acts within the cells and tissues of its origin. These effects are not abolished by histamine antagonists, but corticosteroids inhibit histamine formation by reducing the activity of the enzyme histidine decarboxylase. These observations are relevant to the failure of antihistamines in the treatment of cluster headache, whereas corticosteroids are often effective.

4. *Tyramine.* Tyramine is said to be implicated in the pathogenesis of dietary migraine. It is present in cheese, other dairy products and in some wines. After a tyramine load migraine subjects excrete more free and less conjugated tyramine in the urine than non-migrainous controls. Tyramine releases a number of biogenic monoamines, including catecholamines from sympathetic nerve endings and, perhaps more significantly, serotonin from platelets.

The role of tyramine in dietary migraine was questioned by Anthony and Hinterberger (1975). Comparing the urinary excretion of amines during a migraine headache with the amounts excreted before and after the headache, they found a significant fall in the excretion of tyramine and an equally significant rise in the excretion of serotonin. However, these results were obtained from 10 patients with non-dietary migraine. No significant fluctuations in the urinary excretion of adrenaline, noradrenaline and histamine were observed during the headache phase. Plasma serotonin levels were again much lower during headache than in headache free periods. It is suggested, though not yet proven, that this may reflect the releasing effect of tyramine on serotonin storage sites in platelets. Anthony and Hinterberger (1975) go on to draw attention to other studies which show that the effect of tyramine ingestion is equal to that of placebo in patients with a history of dietary migraine. As their own observations are concerned only with the role of endogenous tyramine in patients with non-dietary migraine, their results do not exclude the possibility that tyramine, whether endogenous or increased by foods containing this amine, may play a part in the pathogenesis of migraine headache either directly or by the release of serotonin. Another vasoactive amine, beta phenylethylamine, is also thought to contribute to the causation of dietary migraine. A possible deficiency of a conjugating enzyme involved in the metabolism of tyramine, as well as a decrease in phenylethylamine oxidizing ability in persons subject to dietary migraine, were reported by Sandler and his collaborators (1974).

Vasoactive Polypeptides

These polypeptides, which are made up of fewer than 100 amino acids, have effects on smooth muscle which are not mediated by alpha and beta receptor pathways. As they have some influence on the tone and calibre of blood vessels their role in the pathogenesis of migraine has been investigated.

1. *Angiotensin.* Angiotensin, formed from renin, stimulates all the muscle walls of the microcirculation and causes vasoconstriction. It is also known to modify adrenergic function via a neurogenic mechanism. However, there is no experimental or clinical evidence that angiotensin is involved in the causation of migraine.

2. *Bradykinin.* Bradykinin is a potent vasodilating polypeptide found in blister fluid and in inflammatory exudates. It is probably both formed and inactivated in the capillary bed and has a half-life of only 20 seconds. It is more potent than histamine in dilating intracranial vessels in man. Bradykinin is present in the subcutaneous tissue fluid of the scalp on the side of hemicrania. If it has any role in migraine, it is only as a locally vasodilating and pain producing agent.

3. *Neurokinin.* Neurokinin may be a mixture of a polypeptide and a proteolytic enzyme. It was first found in the oedema fluid in the scalp during an attack of migraine and was called "headache substance" by Chapman *et al.* (1960). The ability of neurokinin to induce vasodilation and to lower the pain threshold was never confirmed. Like bradykinin, at most, it would have only a local effect.

The kinins appear to originate locally from blood and tissue fluid. There is no good evidence that they have a primary role in the pathogenesis of migraine. It is not even certain that they play a minor part in the causation of local vasodilation and pain.

Lipids

1. *Prostaglandins.* Prostaglandins are unsaturated fatty acids, synthesized in the tissues from arachidonic acid. They are widely distributed in the body and are released in response to both nerve and chemical stimulation. Individual prostaglandins have different effects on the vascular system and their effects also vary with the animal species.

The intravenous infusion of prostaglandin E_1 into healthy subjects produces flushing of the skin and a severe migraine-like headache. It is thought that serotonin can release or activate prostaglandins which then contribute to the vasodilation and aggravate the clinical symptoms of a migraine attack (Anthony, 1972a). However, plasma levels of prostaglandins do not appear to change during a migraine headache. They are difficult to measure because they have a short half-life of less than 30 seconds.

Recent hypotheses propose that the prostaglandins may be modulators of adrenergic neurotransmission in blood vessels and that they may also sensitize responses to other pain producing stimuli (Fozard and Schnieden, 1972).

2. *Free Fatty Acids (FFA).* Plasma free fatty acids (FFA) have recently come under scrutiny when it was found that they rise in the plasma during a migraine headache simultaneously with a fall in plasma serotonin. Once again it is significant that plasma FFA levels do not rise during cluster headache. It is possible that their increase at the time of a migraine headache is a consequence of the release of either serotonin or of prostaglandin E_1.

Estimation of individual FFAs in the plasma has shown that linoleic acid rises most during a migraine headache. Linoleic acid was shown to release platelet serotonin both *in vitro* and *in vivo* in migrainous and in normal subjects. It is also the precursor of prostaglandins in the body and it may be a source of increased prostaglandin E_1 synthesis (Anthony, 1978). These observations permit the speculation that linoleic acid or one of the other FFAs of small molecular size could be the obscure serotonin-releasing factor in plasma. The reduction in circulating levels of serotonin inhibits vascular tone and the added vasodilating effect of prostaglandin E_1 results in the abnormal distension of branches of the carotid arteries which finds its clinical expression in headache.

Steroid Hormones

Some of these hormones, including hydrocortisone, progesterone and 17 beta-oestradiol are known to potentiate responses to adrenaline and noradrenaline, either by inhibiting the inactivating enzyme catechol-o-methyl transferase or by interfering with the uptake of high concentrations of adrenaline or noradrenaline. As yet we have no definite evidence for a role of these steroid hormones in the abnormal vascular reactivity in migraine, but their influence on vasoactive amines could make them a rewarding subject of further study (Fozard and Schnieden, 1972).

Conclusions

The brief review of physiological and biochemical events which may be contributing to the pathogenesis of migraine represents only a minute fraction of the vast volume of experimental work published on these subjects. The references were selected mainly from important original observations and from review articles. It is beyond the scope of this book to cite all references to original research work; many of these will be found in the literature references provided in some of the publications quoted.

The basic cause of migraine remains an enigma, but we shall attempt to construct a very tentative working hypothesis from the mass of complex and often confusing data which we have reviewed.

Widely accepted factors which are important in the pathogenesis of common and classic migraine include the following.

1. An abnormal reactivity of the intracranial and extracranial vessels produces most of the clinical manifestations of migraine. The intracranial arteries constrict while the extracranial arteries dilate. With the exception of the uncommon cases of "symptomatic" migraine, no structural cerebral pathology can be demonstrated.

2. The microcirculation behaves independently from the larger vessels: arterioles and capillaries may constrict while larger arteries dilate. This may lead to the formation of arteriovenous shunts.

3. There is a temporary fall in intracranial perfusion and a later increase in extracranial blood flow during different phases of a migraine attack. Both occur biiaterally, but are more pronounced on the side which corresponds to the patient's symptoms.

4. The sympathetic nervous system does not exert a major influence on the calibre of cranial vessels, but may have an indirect effect on their reactivity to chemical vasoactive agents by setting the tone of the muscular walls of these vessels.

5. The significant fall of plasma serotonin during the headache phase of a migraine attack causes distension of the artery and constriction of the capillaries of the scalp.

Pathogenetic factors which are well supported by experimental evidence, but which are still the subject of controversy, include the following.

1. A permanent abnormality of the platelet membrane of migraine subjects. Platelets aggregate more readily and this contributes to wider fluctuations in plasma serotonin levels.

2. A serotonin releasing substance in the plasma during a migraine attack. The nature of this substance is undetermined, but it is known to be of low molecular weight. Plasma free fatty acids are under scrutiny.

3. Constriction of the microcirculation in the scalp may be enhanced by the direct action of other vasoactive chemical agents. The nature of most of these agents is still obscure.

4. The sensitivity of cranial vessels to serotonin and, perhaps, to other vasoactive substances differs from the sensitivity of other blood vessels in the body. This explains why migraine affects mainly the cranial circulation.

5. Abnormalities in the binding of vasoactive substances to the arterial wall could account for the localization of a migraine headache and for the development of migraine after trauma to extracranial vessels.

6. The local release of circulating vasoactive and pain-producing substances, perhaps including kinins and prostaglandins, contributes to the sterile inflammation of the distended extracranial arterial wall.

All the factors mentioned above can be considered only in the pathogenesis

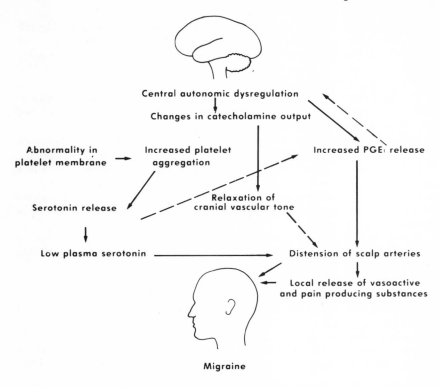

Central autonomic dysregulation

Changes in catecholamine output

Abnormality in
platelet membrane

Increased platelet
aggregation

Increased PGE₁ release

Serotonin release

Relaxation of
cranial vascular tone

Low plasma serotonin

Distension of scalp arteries

Local release of vasoactive
and pain producing substances

Migraine

Fig. 3. Some physiological and biochemical mechanisms involved in the pathogenesis of migraine headache.

of headache and of the focal cerebral symptoms of a migraine attack. The mechanisms causing associated gastrointestinal and other autonomic disorders still await elucidation.

The concept of autonomic dysregulation, though it cannot be defined in terms of specific neural and chemical events, deserves consideration as a primary trigger for the complex multitude of cranial vascular and biochemical changes observed during a migraine attack. Vasoactive agents, such as serotonin and prostaglandins, initially released by autonomic neural impulses, may, in turn, have a modulating effect on central vasomotor and other autonomic nuclei. In this manner, a chain of events which influences both cranial vascular calibre and the activity of the gastrointestinal system is initiated and maintained. The hypothalamus and autonomic nervous system are known to react to stress and to some other environmental triggers which are important at least in the genesis of common migraine. Some of the known physiological and biochemical mechanisms involved in the pathogenesis of migraine headache are summarized in Fig. 3.

It is tempting to suggest that defective central autonomic regulation as well as disordered cranial vascular reactivity and permanent abnormalities in the platelet membrane may be inherited in patients with "genetic" migraine.

Chapter 4

Clinical Features of Migraine and its Variants

Before we consider the specific clinical characteristics of each variety of vascular headache of migraine type we must point out that an individual patient may suffer from more than one type of migraine at different times. The recurrent and paroxysmal occurrence of headache, with or without associated visual or neurological symptoms, is the essential criterion for a diagnosis of migraine. In some patients migraine alternates with muscle contraction (tension) headache and it may not be easy to define the diagnostic borders of each condition clearly. The concept of "tension vascular headache" helps to resolve this dilemma and provides a guideline for the appropriate therapeutic approach.

Common Migraine

The term "common" simply implies that this is by far the most prevalent variety of the migraine syndrome. Common migraine is defined as a vascular headache without striking prodromal or associated symptoms of cerebral dysfunction. It is less often unilateral than classic or complicated migraine and it is more under the influence of precipitating circumstances in the external or internal environment. The popular terms of "sick", "weekend", "menstrual" or "hunger" headache are synonymous with common migraine.

The high frequency of attacks in many sufferers accounts for more misery and interference with the patients' work and enjoyment of life than all the other types of migraine put together. Considering the high prevalence of migraine in the population (5% to 10%), we must agree with Graham (1968) that "the days lost, the children silenced, the husbands angered, the engagements cancelled, the misunderstandings created by this vicious affliction may well top all other human ailments".

In a series of 290 migraine patients from whom detailed histories were available, 231 (79.6%) were diagnosed as suffering from common migraine because they had never experienced major visual disturbances (hemianopia or scotomata) or focal cerebral symptoms before or during the headache (Selby and Lance, 1960). As these patients had been referred to a specialist neurological clinic it is likely that the sample is biased and includes a higher proportion of cases of severe and classic migraine than would be seen by a primary physician. Although no epidemiological data are available, it is more likely that common migraine accounts for about 90% of all patients suffering from vascular headaches of the migraine type.

As mentioned in the first chapter, migraine begins before the age of 40 years in at least 90% of patients. In about one-fifth of these, the first attack is likely to be experienced during the first decade of life, while an onset after the age of 50 years is uncommon. The frequency and severity of attacks of common migraine tend to abate after the age of 50 years, but an occasional recurrence will remind elderly persons of the misery they were prone to during their youth. The abatement of the condition with advancing age occurs equally in both sexes and cannot be attributed entirely to hormonal changes of the menopause. However, not all patients enjoy a spontaneous amelioration as they grow older. The opposite may be true in women approaching the menopause and migraine can occur in both sexes with the development of hypertension or during an intercurrent affective disorder.

The high frequency of attacks is one of the characteristics which distinguish common migraine from other variants of the syndrome. Over one-half of patients suffer from one to four headaches per month; a lower frequency of less than 12 episodes during a year is reported by only 10% to 15% of patients, while some 30% to 35% of the population with common migraine have their lives handicapped by attacks which recur up to three times during a week. The number of headaches in an individual patient will vary not only from year to year, but also at different times of a year depending on environmental circumstances.

The reaction to exogenous or endogenous triggers is another criterion which distinguishes common migraine from the other variants of the syndrome. Many, but by no means all headaches develop after exposure to external stimuli including stress, glare, climatic changes, certain foods and hunger. It is unusual for only a single, specific trigger to elicit an attack on every occasion. A combination of circumstances, such as the stress of preparing a dinner party and the drinking of a glass of red wine during the premenstrual days, will almost certainly provoke an attack on the next day. Premenstrual and menstrual migraine as well as "weekend" and "relaxation" headaches are almost always of the common type. Common migraine is the product of patients' heredity and constitution and of their reaction to exogenous or endogenous events which do not affect a non-migrainous person. A past history of bilious attacks in childhood or of travel sickness, a propensity to dizzy spells and fainting, abnormal vascular responses of the limbs and dysmenorrhoea are indicators of a more widespread constitutional dysfunction of the autonomic nervous system.

Although stress is often the most important cause of a temporary increase in the frequency and severity of migraine headache, it is certainly not a primarily psychogenic illness. This erroneous concept in the mind of the public, held particularly by those who have never suffered from migraine, may have been created by stories in some popular novels of the heroine who manages to avoid an unpleasant situation by having an attack of "migraine" or "vapours". On the contrary, migraine initiated by stress may prevent sufferers from attending to duties and achieving goals, thus setting up a further stress reaction which perpetuates the headache. This may eventually result in the fortunately rare condition of "migraine status" where attacks follow each other at such frequent intervals that the sufferer hardly enjoys a day's freedom over periods which may extend to several weeks or months. This condition can lead to a state of general, severe debility with anorexia, weight loss, sleeplessness and depression; it shows that migraine is by no means always a minor malady. The effects of large amounts of medication add to the patient's ill health; in fact, ergotamine abuse is one of the major causes of migraine status. The long persistence of headache in response to stress may also be created by the coexistence of migraine with psychogenic muscle contraction headache. In some of these cases the excessive contraction of posterior cervical and scalp muscles may be produced or at least aggravated by the initial migrainous vascular headache.

On the other hand, a particularly severe and protracted attack may be followed by an unusually long remission occurring quite independently of treatment. This sequence of events is comparable to the behaviour of some epileptic patients, although the concept of a post-ictal inhibition of hyperexcitable epileptic neurons can hardly be applied to the pathogenetic mechanisms of migraine.

The duration of an attack of common migraine ranges from a few hours to several days. In about two-thirds of patients the headache lasts for less than a day; in only one-sixth it continues for 24 to 48 hours and in the remaining one-sixth it lasts longer than 48 hours. Many headaches begin when the patient first wakes in the morning; others start at the end of a stressful day. It is unusual for the headache to interfere with sleep except in very severe and prolonged episodes.

The drama of a migraine attack unfolds in three acts. This applies equally to common and classic migraine, though in the latter the events during the first act are more spectacular. In common migraine the prodromal phase (first act) usually begins in the late afternoon or evening. The characteristic symptoms vary widely from patient to patient and an individual can experience a varying constellation of symptoms on different occasions. Some of the prodromal complaints are influenced by environmental circumstances which have contributed to the development of an attack. Excessive physical or emotional fatigue or a mood of depression are frequent precursors of the headache. However, the opposite may apply and the patient learns to recognize an unusual capacity for work which can be performed more speedily and efficiently, and a feeling of exhilaration and euphoria as forerunners of a headache on the following morning. Excessive yawning is the specific warning for some people that the next day will be disrupted by headache. These changes in mood and mental alacrity are much more prolonged and less succinct than the premonitory symptoms during the first act of classic migraine. They cannot be attributed to constriction of cerebral vessels and their causal mechanisms are difficult to explain. Conceivably, they may be related to changes in the activity and metabolism of monoamines in the brain, as it is well known that some of these amines are involved in the pathogenesis of depression and in the action of some antidepressant drugs. During the period of excessive mental and physical fatigue, but not during feelings of exhilaration and high intellectual performance, the patient may be aware of a slight, dull or "muzzy" headache which is not severe enough to require analgesic treatment.

The second act of the drama often begins early the next morning when the patient wakes with a more definite, though usually mild, headache which can be either bilateral or unilateral. The situation of the headache may vary in different attacks. In the series of 500 patients reported by Selby and Lance (1960), 191 patients (38%) reported pain all over the head (holocrania) in all their attacks. In a similar proportion of patients, the pain was always hemicranial, though in some 45% of these patients it alternated from side to side in the same or different migraine attacks. During the course of a single attack, whether mild or severe, the pain may change from one side to the other, or an initial hemicrania later develops into a holocrania. However, a generalized migraine headache only rarely later becomes restricted to one side of the head.

As the day advances the headache becomes progressively more intense and the patient may then be confined to bed. It is described as a throbbing or burning pain and some patients are convinced that it must arise from within their cranium. Any movement of the head or body, any cough or jolt, even the slightest motion of the bed such as that created by the steps of others in the room tends to aggravate the pain. The children are ordered to be silent and flowers have to be removed as patients become as intolerant to noise and to odours as they are to light. The blinds are drawn because photophobia is a prominent feature of most migraine attacks in about four-fifths of patients. The patient forgoes breakfast and does not eat for the remainder of the day. Nausea often accompanies the headache. Vomiting may occur within an hour of the headache beginning or much later in the course of the attack. If vomiting occurs frequently, it becomes dry retching; this combines with the intense pain in the head to produce the severe prostration and misery which are the tragic climax of the second act of our migraine drama. While a history of nausea was obtained from 87% of our patients, vomiting occurred in a little more than half (Selby and Lance, 1960). In a few migraineurs, a bout of vomiting signifies a marked reduction in the severity, or even the termination, of the headache. Therefore, some of these people will deliberately induce vomiting to get relief from pain.

The disordered function of the autonomic nervous system can also find its clinical expression in diarrhoea and polyuria. Almost three-quarters of migraine subjects complain of dizziness which may persist for the entire duration of the headache. They describe this as a feeling of lightheadedness — not as true rotational vertigo, though the latter may occur in basilar migraine. Thought processes are retarded, mental concentration and memory are impaired, speech is slow and words may be hard to find while the headache is severe. Mild, vague and diffuse blurring of vision is not unusual during the headache phase of common migraine, particularly if photophobia is pronounced. This blurring may persist for several hours (while the headache is severe) and is quite different to the transient scotomata which characterize classic migraine.

Occasionally, the forehead is flushed and hot on the side of a hemicrania; more often, the face is pale and cold due to the constriction of the microcirculation of the scalp. The branches of one or both superficial temporal arteries may be visibly distended and are almost always tender to pressure or rubbing. Tenderness of the scalp frequently extends over the entire hemicranium. This tenderness of scalp vessels and an aversion to light when the physician attempts to examine the optic fundi or pupils are the only abnormal signs which can be found on examination of the patient during an attack. If the headache is very intense, the secondary contraction of posterior cervical muscles can cause some neck rigidity, leading to suspicion of meningitis or subarachnoid haemorrhage.

Towards the end of the day the pain and nausea abate; the patient is left with a feeling of prostration and malaise which is difficult to define, yet characteristic of migraine. At first some water and, later, a small quantity of food can be tolerated. Patients then strive to rise from their beds and attend to some of the essential obligations which had to be neglected earlier in the day. This is the beginning of the third and anti-climactic act of our drama, the post-headache phase. On the following morning a slight "muzzy" discomfort in the head may remain, the scalp vessels may still be a little tender, mental and physical activities will probably not be quite up to par and working efficiency is likely to be reduced. There is little desire to go shopping or to attend to social commitments. Just as some people feel exhilarated during the prodromal phase, a feeling of exuberance and overwhelming relief that the attack is over may characterize the post-headache phase. Such people will quickly return to their busy schedules and will soon make up both the obligations and pleasures missed during the headache.

Of course, there is an infinite number of variations on the theme of an attack of severe common migraine as described above. Often, the headache begins without any premonitory warning whatever. The severity of pain and the occurrence of nausea and vomiting vary from attack to attack. With appropriate treatment a majority of patients remain able to perform their duties, whether they be domestic, skilled or unskilled, at a slower pace and at a reduced level of efficiency. About one in every five patients never complains of photophobia and at least three out of five patients retain normal vision. Mild attacks are usually short and accompanied by only minor gastrointestinal and vasomotor disorders. At the other end of the spectrum a patient may remain incapacitated and bedridden for several days. The severity of nausea, vomiting and dizziness is proportional to the intensity and duration of the headache.

Vasomotor instability, which is the cause of dizziness, combined with fluid and electrolyte depletion due to vomiting can cause patients to lose consciousness for short periods — usually when they rise from their beds to make their way to the bathroom. The term migraine syncope has been applied to these blackouts during which the patient is pale and sometimes clammy and the limbs are flaccid and motionless. Biting of the tongue, foaming at the mouth and sphincter relaxation do not occur. Consciousness is generally regained within a minute. If syncope is exceptionally severe, mild rigidity and twitching movements of the limbs may be observed. The borderlines between severe syncope and mild epilepsy are not well defined.

In women, if we follow the natural history of common migraine during the lifespan of an individual, we may find that the genetic seeds of the malady are sown by her migrainous mother before she leaves the womb. In early childhood she is described as a "delicate" child, unduly prone to bilious attacks and travel sickness. At school she complains of occasional headaches either during the stress of examinations or after playing games in the sun. These headaches become more pronounced at the time of her menarche and before she is 20 years old they often occur during the premenstrual days. She also suffers from dysmenorrhoea, and her hands and feet react excessively to cold weather. The migraines become more severe when she starts a new job or is distraught by a broken romance. The preparations for her wedding are interrupted by more migrainous episodes, but her fears that the wedding and honeymoon may be marred by headache are often unfounded. During pregnancy she enjoys a complete respite, but her migraine increases again with the interruption of sleep and constant responsibility of looking after her child. Over the next 25 years a fairly predictable pattern of migraine attacks continues. She cannot avoid all the triggers which contribute to them; a temporary aggravation may follow a rather trivial head injury. At the time of the menopause and with the development of hypertension by the age of 50 years, the headaches occur more often, but are less intense and are less often accompanied by vomiting and prostration than they were during her younger years. At the age of 60, when the patient has become adapted to her new lifestyle and has relinquished most of her demanding responsibilities, her migraine improves at last. She enjoys long intervals of freedom and recurrences are provoked mainly by anxieties about her family's welfare.

As will be shown later in this chapter the natural history of common migraine is entirely different from that of other migraine variants.

Classic Migraine

This condition is defined as recurrent, periodic headache which is preceded or accompanied by transient visual, sensory, motor, or other focal cerebral symptoms. It shares many clinical features with common migraine, but there are significant differences which distinguish the two conditions. If we return to our concept of migraine as a drama in three acts, the events during the first act (prodromal phase) are much more dramatic, succinct and shorter in classic migraine, whereas pain and the associated symptoms of autonomic dysfunction of the second act (headache phase) are generally of less intensity and of shorter duration than in common migraine. The third act (post-headache phase) may not take place at all.

The prevalence of *pure* classic migraine has been estimated as being only 10% to 15% of the entire spectrum of the migraine syndrome. This proportion increases if we include the not insignificant number of patients who experience both classic and common migraine. A person with a history of a few attacks of classic migraine during youth may go on to have more frequent episodes of the common type later in life; rarely, the converse may apply. It is not unusual for patients with a long history of common migraine to experience occasional attacks where the headache is preceded or accompanied by visual or focal cerebral symptoms which can create considerable anxiety, particularly on their first appearance.

It is generally thought that a positive family history of migraine can be obtained more often from patients with the classic type, though a few authors claim that the opposite is true. The proportion of female sufferers is lower in classic migraine than in common migraine and there is no significant increase in prevalence during the reproductive years. Environmental circumstances are far less important, but not entirely insignificant, in precipitating attacks of classic migraine and a major proportion of episodes occur "out of the blue".

The onset is usually during adolescence and puberty and *pure* classic migraine tends to abate by the age of 40 years; however, a few patients may continue to experience only the prodromal symptoms, without an ensuing headache.

The frequency of attacks is usually less than 10 a year and may be as low as one to three during a year, with intervals between attacks often exceeding 12 months. This contrasts with the much higher frequency of episodes of common migraine. The duration of attacks also tends to be shorter, rarely exceeding eight to 12 hours.

The clinical features of classic migraine are described below under separate headings, each dealing with the specific visual or cerebral symptoms which characterize the attack. However, it must be emphasized that disorders of sight occur in most patients together with focal neurological disturbances during the prodromal phase. Symptoms such as paraesthesia, a feeling of heaviness of the limbs, or a hesitancy of speech tend to appear a few minutes after normal visual function becomes deranged.

French neurologists regard *migraine ophtalmique* as synonymous with classic migraine and consider all the focal neurological symptoms of a migraine attack under the heading of *migraine accompagnée* or "complicated migraine". The general opinion is that these focal symptoms, whether retinal or cerebral, result from vascular constriction.

Visual Symptoms

A remarkable and interesting variety of visual disturbances is the most important and most widely studied aspect of classic migraine. The disturbances can result from spasm of retinal arteries, which, of course, are branches of the carotid arterial tree, or from transient ischaemia of the occipital lobes or from any part of the optic radiation due to intracranial arterial constriction. The severity and duration of this vasoconstriction and of the consequent localized arteriovenous shunts determine the nature and duration of the visual disorder. Most often, the disturbances last from 10 to 30 minutes and occur during the prodromal phase before the headache begins; however, they may occasionally appear or recur at the height of a headache and, rarely, as it abates.

On clinical grounds, it is not always possible to decide whether the symptoms are due to ischaemia of the retina or of the central optic pathway, or both. In both situations a mild reduction of perfusion can produce "positive" symptoms, such as flashing or scintillating lights or figures, or "negative" symptoms, which include patchy or diffuse scotomata or various defects of the visual fields. It is assumed that the "positive" symptoms are the expression of abnormal stimulation of retinal or cerebral neurons, while the "negative" symptoms are produced by their inhibition, which is the outcome of a more severe degree of ischaemia.

If the visual disturbances are confined to the field of one eye they must arise from the retina; bilateral scotomata, whether patchy or diffuse, are also attributed to reduced retinal perfusion. The central visual pathways, particularly the occipital lobes, are implicated if either "positive" or "negative" visual phenomena have a hemianopic distribution.

The pattern of visual symptoms is stereotyped only in a minority of patients. In most, both what is seen or not seen, as well as the part of the visual field

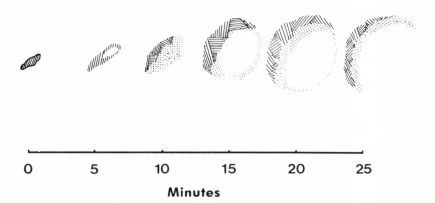

0   5   10   15   20   25

Minutes

Fig. 4. Pattern of scotoma (dots) and of a shimmering crescent (cross-hatched) during the visual aura timed and drawn by a patient who had similar visual symptoms with each attack.

involved, tend to change from attack to attack. The most common "positive" symptoms described are bright, scintillating lights which can appear as crescents or flashes moving from one side of the visual field to the other (Fig. 4). Bright spots or spheres and different geometric shapes (particularly zig-zag lines which can be white or coloured) are frequently reported. The pattern of the wall of a fortress viewed from above (from which the terms fortification spectra and teichopsia are derived) is relatively uncommon. On the other hand, the disorder of vision can be more diffuse and patients often report that everything they look at appears "as though seen through a sheet of rippling water".

The following case history, provided by a highly intelligent woman of 35 years, is a good example of classic migraine with both "positive" and "negative" visual symptoms during the aura.

The attacks began when she was only six years old. They were frequent during childhood, but in adult life she averaged no more than one or two per year. The first premonition consisted of "fireworks" seen before either the right or left eye; these soon gave way to grey or green "snakes" wriggling before both eyes. Next, her vision became blurred and she could discern only parts of objects she looked at. Sometimes these objects looked strange and assumed wrong dimensions. On occasions she felt that one hand, always on the same side as the ensuing hemicrania, did not belong to her "as if it were somebody else's hand". The headache came on after varying intervals ranging from 10 minutes to two hours from the onset of premonitory visual symptoms. It was always hemicranial, involving either the right or left side, and was accompanied by intense photophobia and vomiting.

Loss of vision of varying extent and severity can appear as the visual "hallucinations" subside or may occur *ab initio*. Many patients report patchy scotomata, or holes in their vision when parts of near or distant objects they look at are either blurred or cannot be seen at all. A patch of several lines on a page of print disappears; these patches often have an irregular shape with a zig-zag border. In others, the scotoma, whether monocular or binocular, is more diffuse, but of varying density. In a few patients, vision is lost completely in one or both eyes for a short period. Such disturbing events create great anxiety for the patient, particularly at the first occurrence. Central vision alone is lost in some attacks, while others clearly describe a partial or complete defect confined to the periphery of the visual field of one or both eyes. In general, this great variety of scotomata is explained more easily on the basis of retinal rather than occipital lobe ischaemia.

An example of classic migraine with a purely visual, and presumably retinal, aura is provided by the following case history.

A motor mechanic, aged 44 years, with a history of tension headaches since youth, had begun to suffer from classic migraine at the age of 42 years. The attacks occurred at intervals of from two to four months and were not related to any environmental circumstances. Each attack was heralded by visions of shimmering, wavy lines before both eyes, followed by bilateral patchy scotomata. These visual disorders persisted for periods ranging from 30 to 60 minutes. As his vision returned to normal either a generalized or a left hemicranial headache came on and progressively increased in severity. It was accompanied by photophobia, nausea, occasional vomiting and by tenderness of his scalp.

Cerebral disorders of vision occur less often, but are even more varied and fascinating than those we have ascribed to a retinal aetiology. They are generally hemianopic disturbances and the side of the hemianopia can change from attack to attack. It may extend across one field into the other; in rare instances the hemianopia is bitemporal. More often, the upper or lower halves of both fields are involved and such an "altitudinal" hemianopia is almost pathognomonic of migraine. We can only speculate whether it results from ischaemia above or below the calcarine cortex of both occipital lobes, or from reduced perfusion of the upper or lower halves of both retinae. Either hypothesis would serve.

At times the hemianopic defect is confined to central vision. This is exemplified by the following case.

A man of 51 experienced three episodes of central vision disturbance over a period of 18 months. In the third, he suddenly found himself unable to see the second half of each word or paragraph (that is, the right half of the paper) he was trying to read. This defect did not extend into his peripheral visual field. Clear colourless shimmers were confined to the lower half of the right central visual field. His sight returned to normal within 30 minutes; he then had a mild transfrontal headache without associated nausea. One of the preceding two episodes consisted of a similar right hemianopia confined to central vision; in the second, he saw shimmers before both eyes, but could not localize them precisely. The duration of visual disturbance was about 30 minutes for each attack. Full neurological examination was unrewarding and electroencephalographic examination some four months after the last episode showed normal results.

Cortical visual disorders similar to those of presumed retinal origin, comprise symptoms which can be explained on the basis of either neuronal excitation or inhibition. The visual hallucinations, which may be "unformed" or "formed" have aroused considerable interest and speculation in neurological literature. The most informative detail is contained in the descriptions from physicians who personally experienced these visual phenomena. They are of infinite variety — coloured or transparent, ranging from irregular or regular geometric forms to the most complex, and, at times, consist of bizarre visions of people and complete scenarios with distorted spatial relationships.

Geometric shapes far outnumber the more fascinating "formed" visions and, again, bright, crescent shapes, often with a jagged medial edge and confined to one half of the visual field, are most commonly described. These shapes tend to move slowly across the half field of vision, either from the periphery to the centre or in the opposite direction. Their rate of movement in some well documented cases agrees with the speed of the "spreading depression of Leão" which was referred to in the previous chapter. As the visual hallucination (stimulation) is often followed by impairment or loss of vision (inhibition) in the same part of the visual field, it is postulated that a wave of cortical depression consequent to excessive stimulation is the responsible pathogenetic mechanism.

In a few cases where an electroencephalogram (EEG) was recorded while a patient suffered a migrainous cortical visual aura the tracing contained focal slow wave abnormalities consistent with the side of the hemianopia. In other cases, the EEG abnormality, though mainly post-central, was bilateral. More recently, computerized tomographic (CT) brain scans were obtained from a few migrainous patients during or soon after a cortical visual aura. Some of these showed areas of dimished density, surrounded by oedema, from the appropriate cortical region. Both the EEG and CT scan abnormalities diminished or disappeared within a few days. They will receive more attention in Chapter 5.

It is not surprising that the visual disturbances of cortical origin are often accompanied by other focal cerebral symptoms during the aura of classic migraine. The following case history illustrates this.

A 29-year-old woman had suffered from both classic and common migraine since childhood. The attacks of classic migraine occurred at infrequent and irregular intervals and were usually heralded by an aura of flickering "neon" lights in the right visual field. These persisted for from 15 to 30 minutes. During that time, the patient usually experienced numbness of the right half of the face and lips; the numbness would then spread to the right hand and arm, but only rarely into the leg. As the visual and sensory symptoms subsided, a predominantly right hemicrania developed with increasing severity and was accompanied by intense photophobia and vomiting. On the other hand, the headache of her attacks of common migraine was usually felt over the left hemicranium.

It should be noted that in this patient the visual and sensory disturbances were on the same side of the body as the ensuing headache. This is not an uncommon occurrence and permits a confident diagnosis of classic rather than symptomatic migraine due to an underlying cerebral vascular malformation.

If the area of ischaemia extends forward to the parietal lobe, patients may experience rather bizarre visual distortions, including micropsia or macropsia, where part or all of their environment suddenly and temporarily looks either abnormally small or large. The zenith of formed visual hallucinations of a very complex nature is to be found in the writings and drawings of the nun Hildegard of Bingen (1098-1180) which have been interpreted as indisputably migrainous (Sacks, 1971). The fact that Hildegard was a mystic and a highly imaginative writer may help to explain why the majority of our patients do not describe similar experiences.

Disorders of ocular movement causing a transient and usually brief diplopia, which may be horizontal or vertical, occur infrequently during the premonitory phase of a migraine attack. The appearance of this diplopia before the headache begins, its brief duration and the absence of an obvious squint distinguish it from ophthalmoplegic migraine where ocular muscle palsies persist for long periods and diplopia may even be permanent. This condition will be discussed later under the topic of ophthalmoplegic migraine.

Temporary inequality in the size of the pupil and a mild ptosis are noted more often than diplopia during an episode of classic migraine. The symptoms usually begin during the premonitory phase and may persist during the headache and for a short time afterwards.

There is an enormous and, at times, confusing literature on the diverse visual disorders which individual patients can experience during classic migraine. They can arouse fears of strokes and of brain tumours in the minds of some patients. Therefore, it is important for the primary physician to recognize them as a characteristic feature of the migraine syndrome and to reassure patients without involving them in invasive or costly investigations.

Sensory Symptoms

Focal sensory symptoms are less common than disorders of vision in patients with classic migraine. From several reports in the literature, their incidence ranges from 33% to 66% of attacks. They consist mainly of subjective sensations of numbness or of tingling and pins and needles. Similar to the visual disorders, they occur predominantly during the prodromal phase, but they may come on simultaneously with the headache, or later, at its peak. In general, the sensory disturbances last for 10 to 30 minutes; if they occur during the aura they tend to abate before the onset of pain.

Numbness and paraesthesia are felt predominantly in the fingers and may then ascend to the hand and forearm. Without involving the upper arm or shoulder, they often spread to the lips, either ipsilateral to the hand or on both sides. A circumoral sensation of numbness, extending into both sides of the tongue, is often described. The side of the nose and the face are usually spared. The trunk and lower limbs are much less often affected than the hands and lips.

The march of dysaesthesia from fingers to lips is slower than the progression of a focal sensory epileptic seizure. It is traditionally attributed to ischaemia of the sensory cortex, the paraesthesia indicating stimulation and the numbness inhibition. The relatively large area of the sensory cortex devoted to fingers, lips and tongue would support a cortical localization. Bruyn (1968) has chosen the term "cheiro-oral syndrome" to describe the finger-lip-tongue distribution of dysaesthesia and considers that they may originate in sensory nuclei of the thalamus rather than in the sensory cortex. More than one-half of his series of patients felt the focal sensory symptoms on the side contralateral to the hemicrania; in about one-third they were on the same side and in the remaining one-sixth they were bilateral. In my own experience, ipsilateral paraesthesia outnumbers a contralateral distribution. A history of sensory symptoms on the *same* side as hemicrania is a reliable clue to a diagnosis of classic rather than symptomatic migraine.

Intense numbness of the fingers and hands naturally impair their use, even if there is no primary interference with motor function. Similarly, speech may become indistinct or lisping may occur if the lips and tongue are numb. Only in rare instances does the dysaesthesia persist beyond an hour; in isolated cases it becomes permanent. These cases will be discussed under the heading of complicated migraine.

If we bear in mind that the pathogenetic mechanism underlying migrainous sensory disturbances is constriction of cerebral vessels, which can be focal or diffuse, it is not surprising that disorders of vision or of speech occur in conjunction with the dysaesthesia in many attacks. The following case history demonstrates this.

A 28-year-old truck driver reported about 12 attacks of migraine over a period of four years. Each began suddenly with numbness and tingling of his right hand which rapidly ascended to the right forearm and then to the right side of the face, particularly the mouth, lips and tongue. The dysaesthesia then passed down into the right side of the chest to the waist, but not into the leg. During the 10 to 15 minutes while he remained aware of the sensory disturbances, he could squeeze or pinch his right fingers without feeling pain. Within seconds after the onset of the sensory symptoms he would find himself unable to use the correct word to express his thoughts, and he often said words different to those he had intended. However, he had no difficulty in understanding what others said to him. At about the same time he noted that objects in his right visual field seemed further away than they actually were; in some attacks there was also a partial restriction of the peripheral part of the right field of vision. The dysaesthesia ceased and his speech and vision returned to normal just before a bifrontal, severe, throbbing headache came on. The pain progressively increased in severity and was accompanied by nausea; it improved gradually after 12 to 36 hours, but the scalp over his forehead remained sore and tender to touch for the next two to three days.

On the few occasions where an opportunity presents to examine patients during the time of their sensory symptoms, an objective impairment in the appreciation of touch or pain stimuli may be found, while proprioception, discriminative sensation and stereognosis are only rarely deficient. This is difficult to explain on the basis of ischaemia confined to the cortical sensory areas and would be consistent with some involvement of the thalamic sensory nuclei.

The diagnosis of migraine presents no problems if a previous history of similar sensory symptoms or of vascular headache can be elicited. If such a history is lacking, both patients and their doctors may be more apprehensive about the possibility of a serious cerebral lesion. This is illustrated by the following case history.

A physician, aged 58 years, had been treated for mild hypertension in the past. While driving to a home consultation, he suddenly became aware of a strange paraesthesia confined to his right hand and forearm. As he could not grip the steering wheel firmly with his hand, he decided to pull up to the kerb. The dysaesthesia recovered within 10 minutes and he was then able to continue his journey. Soon afterwards, when he was examining his patient's abdomen, he could not see clearly and thought that his visual field was restricted. When he returned to his surgery after about 30 minutes a left hemicrania came on and became so intense that he was forced to go home. He felt bilious, but did not vomit. Detailed neurological examination the next day showed no objective sensory impairment, nor any other abnormal signs. His blood pressure was mildly raised. He then recalled two attacks of severe headache during the preceding 10 years; each lasted for about a day and neither was associated with any focal neurological symptoms. Electroencephalographic examination recorded within 24 hours after these disturbing symptoms showed a moderate amount of slow activity of low amplitude from the posterior half of the left cerebral hemisphere.

This physician and his partners had seriously considered a diagnosis of a transient cerebral ischaemic attack. He was reassured that the visual impairment some time after the dysaesthesia had subsided and the later severe and progressive left hemicrania were diagnostic of classic migraine.

Disorders of Movement

While a subjective feeling of heaviness and weakness of an arm or hand often occurs together with dysaesthesia in the same limb, a more severe paresis is a very rare event in classic migraine. It is more likely to appear if the aura is unduly prolonged; in the majority of such cases paresis is confined to the upper limb. The patient is usually also dysphasic if the limb innervated by the dominant cerebral hemisphere is paretic. Examination of the patient during the attack shows only a mild to moderate weakness without increase of muscle tone or exaggerated deep tendon reflexes. Recovery of normal strength within an hour is the rule. The following case history illustrates the clinical features which justify a confident diagnosis of classic migraine.

A woman, aged 30 years, with a history of classic migraine heralded by a visual aura during the preceding 11 years, reported that her left arm suddenly became numb and felt swollen. She was then unable to move this arm. She could not speak at all for some five minutes and afterwards her speech was slow and slurred. She became intensely upset, trembled and hyperventilated. The numbness and paresis of her left upper limb, as well as her speech, recovered completely within 15 minutes. She then developed a severe holocrania and mild photophobia. Her family physician found no objective abnormality when he examined her three hours after the onset of symptoms, which had obviously frightened her very much.

In contrast with the brief duration of weakness in classic migraine there are rare, but well documented, instances of a more dense hemiplegia involving both upper and lower limbs and persisting for several hours or days. We shall discuss this hemiplegic migraine later as one of the varieties of complicated migraine.

It was mentioned earlier in this chapter that both the visual and sensory symptoms of a migraine attack can be attributed either to stimulation or inhibition. Stimulation of the motor cortex would result in focal (partial) seizures. Fortunately, this occurs only very rarely in classic migraine. A few patients refer to mild trembling of one or both arms at the height of an attack, but this is usually due to distress and anxiety.

There are isolated case reports of various involuntary movements, some choreic and others myoclonic, which recurred during each migraine attack. These movements were confined mainly to the face and arm, but their description in papers mostly published more than 50 years ago does not provide sufficient information to justify inclusion of such extrapyramidal movement disorders as a manifestation of classic migraine. Similarly, the very rare occurrence of facial paralysis, which may be of upper or lower motor neuron type, would hardly give it the status of a nosologic entity. This subject is dealt with critically by Bruyn (1968), who points out that recurrent facial palsies in migrainous patients were usually associated with ocular palsies which involved either the right or left side in different attacks.

If we accept the pathogenetic concept of focal or diffuse intracranial vasoconstriction, we must wonder why disorders of movement are so rare in comparison with the frequency of visual and sensory symptoms during a migraine attack.

Speech Disorders

Some of the case histories cited earlier in this chapter made reference to the patients' difficulties with speech. They tend to appear shortly after the onset of visual or sensory symptoms during the migrainous aura. These speech disorders are less prevalent than complaints about disturbed vision or sensation. They are usually mild and short-lasting and may consist of a difficulty either in finding the correct words (dysphasia) or in pronouncing them clearly (dysarthria). Dysphasia is almost always expressive and the writer has no records of patients who were unable to understand what was said to them. They usually describe that they know what they want to say, but are surprised when an entirely wrong word comes out. Speech tends to become slow and hesitant and, less often, stammering. On occasions, in a more prolonged migrainous aura, dysphasia is only part of a more general sense of confusion, difficulty in mental concentration and slowing of thought processes. Dysarthria, due to malfunction of the muscles required for articulation, is less common than dysphasia in migraine. In this condition speech becomes slow and slurred. In the more severe cases, it sounds "jumbled". This slurring of speech can appear when the patient recovers from expressive dysphasia or it may occur simultaneously with it.

If dysphasia is severe or happens to a person without a previous history of migraine, the correct diagnosis may not immediately come to mind.

A lecturer in veterinary science, aged 26, with a history of a few tension headaches, but not of migraine, was riding in a bus when she suddenly could not think of words to express her ideas. After she alighted from the bus, she found that she could not name the things she wanted to buy in a store. Within five to 10 minutes she became aware of numbness which at first involved the entire right hand and later was confined to the ulnar three fingers of this hand. Both the dysphasia and numbness recovered after some 15 minutes; then a predominantly left sided headache appeared and gradually increased in severity. She returned home and went to bed in a darkened room because she was intensely photophobic. On the next day she felt utterly exhausted and had a mild left hemicrania. Neurological and general examinations showed no abnormality; normal EEG and CT brain scan results, obtained seven days later, confirmed that her complaints were not due to structural cerebral pathology.

Various symptoms of disordered function of the temporal or parietal lobes are described by a few patients and occur mainly during severe attacks of classic migraine. They include feelings of depersonalization, *déja vu* experiences, dreamy states, disturbances of body image and a variety of visual distortions. We have referred to some of these in our discussion of the visual prodromata of migraine. These complaints, which may at first sound bizarre, are never stereotyped, but they are often associated with disordered speech or sensory perception.

Vertigo

A broad definition of vertigo is simply "any illusion of movement". Patients may feel either that their environment moves around them or that they themselves are moving in relation to their surroundings. Vertigo results from a disturbance in the labyrinthine end organs or their central connections in the brain stem and cerebellum. It must be clearly distinguished from a sensation of "lightheadedness" which is due to reduced cerebral perfusion and is often described as "dizziness". Most patients regard the terms "dizziness", "giddiness" and "vertigo" as synonymous and a painstaking analysis of their subjective experiences is needed to make a distinction between dizziness and true vertigo. In either condition, an unsteadiness of stance or gait will accompany the subjective experience. For our discussion of specific symptoms associated with different varieties of migraine, a clear distinction between "dizziness" and true "vertigo" is of more than academic importance.

Dizziness, that is, a feeling of lightheadedness and unsteadiness, precipitated or aggravated by rising and stooping, occurs with equal frequency in common and classic migraine. It was reported by some 72% of 131 patients (Selby and Lance, 1960) and usually occurs during the headache and not in the prodromal phase. It is an expression of the vasomotor instability which is so common in migrainous subjects and to which we have referred earlier in this and the previous chapter. If the fall in cerebral perfusion is sufficiently intense and prolonged, consciousness may be lost for a short period; we have already mentioned the concept of migraine syncope in our discussion of common migraine.

Vertigo, on the other hand, is a symptom of classic migraine and occurs mainly during the premonitory phase. An illusion of movement was described by 33% of 217 patients (Selby and Lance, 1960) and in 28% of the series of 150 patients analysed by Klee (1968). This high incidence of vertigo may be largely due to misinterpretation of the histories obtained from patients; many find it difficult to distinguish between lightheadedness and true vertigo. In the migraineurs seen by the author in recent years a history of true vertigo was recorded in less than 10% of cases when this symptom was defined by strict criteria. It is certainly less common than visual or sensory symptoms, but it is more prevalent than disorders of movement.

The duration of vertigo is usually much shorter than that of a visual or sensory aura. On average it lasts only two to three minutes; it may persist for up to 15 minutes on rare occasions. In some migrainous subjects, brief episodes of vertigo occur without ensuing headache, or only a mild, dull discomfort in the head and minimal nausea may be experienced after recovery from giddiness.

The following case history describes events which justify the interpretation of short episodes of vertigo as part of the patient's migraine syndrome.

A 45-year-old man, with a history of classic migraine preceded by a visual aura between the ages of 22 and 29 years, began to experience recurrent attacks of vertigo at the age of 43. He described a subjective sense of rotation of his body and was so unsteady that he preferred to sit down. There was no associated aural discomfort or tinnitus. He felt bilious, but did not vomit. Vertigo persisted for only two to five minutes and was not followed by headache. At the age of 44, while he was broadcasting at a country fair, he suddenly felt pins and needles on the left side of his body, including the face and lips. The paraesthesia lasted for some three minutes and was accompanied by some slurring of his speech. He felt slightly bilious and very exhausted, but he had no headache. Full otological assessment, including audiometry, electronystagmography and caloric testing, provided no definite evidence for a primary or residual labyrinthine disorder. He was mildly hypertensive, but full neurological examination and electroencephalography showed no abnormality. The key to the diagnosis of migrainous vertigo was found in this man's past history of classic migraine and in the single, brief episode of hemiparaesthesia, dysarthria and nausea.

Just as visual hallucinations and scotomata can occur without ensuing headache, it is not unusual for short episodes of vertigo to occur without any associated symptoms in migrainous subjects. The brief duration of vertigo, which is usually less than five minutes, and the absence of deafness, tinnitus and other aural discomfort serve to distinguish this migrainous vertigo from Meniere's syndrome.

Recurrent brief episodes of intense rotational vertigo without headache are so often reported by post-menopausal women with a history of migraine in earlier years that we shall return to this subject later in a discussion of migraine without headache.

As the vertigo we have so far described is not associated with dysarthria, diplopia, or other symptoms of a brain stem dysfunction, it is reasonable to suppose that it arises in the labyrinth and is caused by constriction of the labyrinthine end arteries. As an alternative to "spasm" a reduced perfusion in the vascular territory of the labyrinthine arteries during the phase of generalised vasoconstriction might be considered. There is some clinical evidence to suggest that recurrence of such impaired perfusion can result in permanent damage to the labyrinth, analogous to irreversible retinal or focal cerebral damage in well documented cases of complicated migraine. Some of these patients eventually go on to develop deafness and tinnitus and Symonds (1951) proposes that migraine is one among the many causes of Meniere's syndrome. The recent concept of "secondary labyrinthine hydrops" would now be more appropriate.

While the labyrinth appears to be the seat of the disorder in most cases of vertigo with classic migraine, in some patients a different and wider constellation of symptoms implicates the central labyrinthine connections in the brain stem. A syndrome termed "basilar artery migraine" was described by Bickerstaff (1961, 1962) who had then seen some 30 patients with a similar sequence of symptoms over a period of five years. The clinical features of this syndrome are an onset of visual phenomena, either dimming or loss of vision in part or the whole of both visual fields, or flashes of light which may involve either half or the whole of the field of vision on both sides. These visual disorders are attributed to reduced blood flow in the posterior cerebral arteries, the terminal branches of the basilar artery. Vertigo, unsteadiness of gait and dysarthria follow shortly after the onset of the visual disorder. Some patients also experience bilateral paraesthesia around the mouth and in the hands and feet. The duration of these complaints ranged from 10 to 30 minutes and they were followed by a severe and predominantly occipital headache. About one-third of Bickerstaff's (1962) patients suffered a short disturbance of consciousness without specific phenomena of epilepsy after the visual and neurological symptoms had disappeared and before the headache began. This loss of consciousness, as well as vertigo, ataxia and dysarthria may reasonably be attributed to transient and mild ischaemia of the brain stem including the reticular formation. A similar combination of symptoms is more frequently seen in older patients with transient basilar ischaemia, but usually without the negative or positive visual disturbances. The diagnosis of basilar artery migraine, rather than transient vertebrobasilar ischaemia due to arterial disease, is suggested by the young age of most patients, often by a family history of migraine and by the observation that attacks were either isolated or occurred infrequently against a background of more typical episodes of classic migraine. Severe headache and vomiting, which followed after the dramatic prodromal symptoms, are a further strong argument in favour of a diagnosis of migraine.

I am indebted to Dr P.M. Williamson for the following case history which shows many of the typical features of basilar artery migraine:

A 15-year-old schoolboy with no history of migraine, but with a family history of both common and classic migraine, complained of dimming of vision in his left visual field after a day's surfing. On his way home his gait was very unsteady and he tended to fall to the right. He experienced tingling sensations in all limbs and later had an occipital headache and nausea. He then became progressively more confused and disorientated and lapsed into a state of stupor. On arrival at the hospital he was aroused with some difficulty and complained of severe occipital headache; he vomited twice. He was afebrile, had no neck stiffness and no abnormal neurological signs could be elicited. He was too drowsy to co-operate with testing of his visual fields. After 12 hours he had recovered apart from a mild left hemicrania. Electroencephalography (EEG) recorded on the day after his admission to hospital, showed prominent bilateral post-central delta and theta activity (1Hz-5Hz). This slow activity was no longer evident in a progress tracing obtained three weeks later when the EEG was reported as within normal limits.

Of course, there is no good reason why the basilar artery and its branches should be exempt from the same abnormal constriction which is widely accepted as the basic mechanism of disordered cerebral function in other areas.

In addition to the large variety of visual and neurological symptoms which characterize the attack, the natural history of classic migraine also differs from that of common migraine in many respects. A genetic predisposition is of similar importance in both conditions. A person with pure classic migraine, as distinct from one who suffers from both the classic and common forms of the disease, is usually not a delicate child suffering from bilious attacks and travel sickness during early childhood. The first attack often occurs before the age of 20 years and the frequency of attacks is low, with free intervals ranging from several months to several years. There is no relationship to the menstrual cycle or to pregnancy, though the significance of the latter is difficult to determine because of the long remissions which occur at other times. With occasional exceptions, classic migraine is not influenced by any of the multitude of environmental circumstances which may evoke an attack of common migraine. It is also less dependent on the patient's personality and emotional state. The attacks are not liable to increase with the development of hypertension, nor do they necessarily decrease with advancing age. After middle age there is a tendency for transient visual disorders, vertigo and focal cerebral symptoms to occur without headache. The presumed angiospastic symptoms can hardly ever be influenced by treatment with pharmacological agents, but if appropriate drugs are taken early in the premonitory phase, relief from headache is more often achieved than in common migraine.

Complicated Migraine

In the past the concept of complicated migraine has received more attention from European authors than from American or English writers. We shall use it to distinguish some rare migraine variants where visual or focal neurological disorders outlast the headache and may even persist permanently. Although it is one of the most uncommon components of the migraine syndrome, it is important for physicians to recognize it as such and to explain the implications and prognosis to their patients. The diagnosis can be considered only if the patient has a preceding history of another form of migraine, or if the visual or focal neurological symptoms develop just before, during or after a vascular headache of migraine type.

We have no reliable information on the prevalence or sex incidence of complicated migraine, but we know that genetic factors are important in the aetiology of one form of hemiplegic migraine and that the frequency of attacks is very low in every patient. We shall confine our discussion to four varieties of complicated migraine: visual, ophthalmoplegic, hemiplegic and dysphrenic.

Persistent Defects of Vision

We have mentioned earlier that both the scotomata and hemianopic defects of vision usually persist for no longer than 30 minutes in an attack of classic migraine. The neurological and ophthalmological literature now provides many reports where the visual impairment lasted for weeks or indefinitely. In some of these patients occlusion of the retinal artery, or of one of its branches, could be demonstrated. Not only defects of vision, but also the positive symptoms of shimmering and flickering lights may persist for long periods. Symonds (1951) draws attention to the fact that in his own patients, as well as in others recorded in the literature in adequate detail, the persistent visual disturbance developed after an attack of "classic" migraine in which the usual visual symptoms were not followed by headache. He suggests that in these patients severe vasoconstriction persisted instead of being followed by the usual vasodilation. One of Symonds' (1951) patients complained of a persistent flickering of vision which interfered with, but did not prevent, reading over a period of 15 years. He goes on to show that prolonged arterial spasm can cause not only irreversible damage in the retina, but also in the central visual pathways. He presents the case history of a man, aged 54 years, with a history of classic migraine since childhood. The headache was preceded by rapidly moving wavy lines in either the right or left half of his visual field. At the age of 54 years, he experienced the usual visual aura in his right field of vision. No headache followed, but the vision of wavy lines persisted and became smaller over a period of six months. He was found to have a homonymous right hemianopia with sparing of central vision. Left carotid and vertebral angiography showed no abnormality and excluded an underlying cerebral vascular malformation.

A thorough review of the literature and many illustrative case histories of migrainous patients with persistent defects of vision are available in volume 2 of the third édition of the book *Clinical Neuro-Ophthalmology* by Walsh and Hoyt (1969). They analyse the clinical features which distinguish retinal from cerebral lesions and cite interesting examples of permanent homonymous and often congruous scotómata, which may be single or multiple (Fig. 5.). The ophthalmoscopic evidence of spasm or occlusion of branches of the retinal ar-

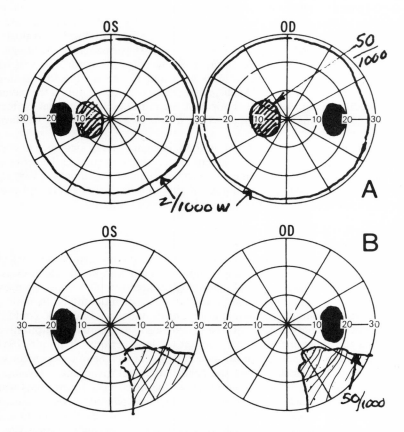

Fig. 5. Persistent defects in the visual field of patients with classic migraine. A. Homonymous left paracentral scotoma. B. Congruous right lower homonymous defect, which remained after a transient episode of right homonymous hemianopia (reproduced from *Clinical Neuro-Ophthalmology*, Vol. 2, 3rd Edition, 1969, by F.B. Walsh and W.F. Hoyt with the permission of the Williams and Wilkins Company).

tery, as well as the recent demonstration of infarcts in the region of the central visual pathways in computerized tomographic brain scans provide the most compelling evidence for retinal or cerebral angiospasm which is so far available.

Ophthalmoplegic Migraine

In this rare variant of migraine the attacks of headache are associated with partial or complete paralyses of the ocular muscles. The oculomotor (third) nerve is selectively involved in almost 90% of cases; an abducens (sixth) nerve palsy comes next in frequency; a few patients have an isolated trochlear (fourth nerve) weakness and very few cases of total ophthalmoplegia have been reported.

Ophthalmoplegic migraine has aroused much interest and controversy for almost a hundred years. Its clear nosological entity as part of the migraine syndrome has been established through the perfection of angiographic techniques during the last four decades. The clinical characteristics which distinguish ophthalmoplegic migraine from other ocular palsies are now well defined.

Friedman *et al.* (1962) found only eight cases of ophthalmoplegic migraine in a total of 5000 migraine patients seen over a period of 30 years. A family history of migraine is not recorded as often as in other forms of this disorder. The first attack usually occurs in childhood or adolescence.

The following clinical criteria suggest a diagnosis of ophthalmoplegic migraine.

1. A preceding history of either common or classic migraine.

2. The headache usually, but not always, precedes ophthalmoplegia. It is often a severe pain felt behind or above the eye; it always occurs on the same side as the ophthalmoplegia. Ptosis is usually noted before paralysis of ocular muscles; in third nerve palsies the pupil is always dilated and fails to react to direct light stimulation. The ocular muscle palsy may be partial or complete and more than one nerve supplying the external ocular muscles can be involved.

3. Although headache can persist for two to three days, ophthalmoplegia always outlasts it; recovery within one to four weeks occurs in the majority of cases.

4. Attacks of ophthalmoplegic migraine tend to recur at irregular, but often long intervals. Both headache and ocular muscle paralysis may switch sides in subsequent attacks. Some patients suffer more than 20 attacks during their life. At times, ophthalmoplegia may appear without headache.

5. If the paralysis is severe, recovery can be incomplete. In rare instances, the patient may be left with a permanent ocular palsy.

The diagnosis of ophthalmoplegic migraine presents no problem if the patient provides a history of one or more similar attacks, particularly if the opposite side was affected on previous occasions. It is impossible to be so confident if the patient is seen at the time of the first attack. Carotid and vertebral arteriography are then essential to exclude an aneurysm of the circle of Willis; the more remote possibilities of diabetes, syphilis, endocrine ophthalmopathy and orbital mucocele must be eliminated by appropriate investigations. Suspicion of an aneurysm is aroused if the patient has no history of migraine, if the third nerve palsy appears without an immediately preceding headache and if all previous ocular muscle pareses affected the same eye. As cerebral arteriography is a safe procedure without undue risk, now it should always be performed to provide a firm diagnosis.

A typical example of ophthalmoplegic migraine is illustrated by the following case history.

A young man, 17 years of age, had experienced an average of four attacks of severe right frontal headache per year since the age of 13 years. The headaches persisted for one to two hours only. They were associated with vomiting, but not with any visual or neurological symptoms. In July, 1979, he again had a right frontal and periorbital headache, which was more intense than on previous occasions and did not respond to analgesic therapy. This time, the headache continued for 24 hours. Some 14 hours after the onset of this headache he noted a right ptosis and complained of diplopia in all directions of gaze. No family history of migraine was recorded. When he was admitted to hospital two days after the onset of this attack, he had a right ptosis of moderate severity. The right pupil was dilated and failed to react to direct and consensual light stimulation. He had a paresis of all muscles supplied by the third cranial nerve. No bruits were audible over the orbits. Neurological examination was otherwise unrewarding; blood pressure was 14.7kPa (110mm Hg) systolic and 9.33kPa (70mm Hg) diastolic. Random plasma glucose ranged from 5.2mmol/L to 8.7mmol/L and a full biochemical profile was unremarkable. Electroencephalography and computerized tomographic brain scan showed no abnormalities. No aneurysm was demonstrated by right carotid and right vertebral arteriograms. There was no other vascular anomaly or displacement of the intracranial vessels. On the day after his admission the right ptosis began to lift, the right pupil reacted sluggishly to light and some recovery of the right third nerve palsy was apparent. When he was discharged from hospital six days later, only a very slight right ptosis and minimal right oculo-motor palsy remained.

The pathogenesis of ophthalmoplegic migraine is still a subject of controversy. The most attractive theories implicate either compression or ischaemia of the oculomotor nerve. This nerve, as well as the nearby fourth and sixth cranial nerves, may be compressed or stretched by the rigid, oedematous wall of a distended internal carotid artery in the cavernous sinus. This arterial distension would also serve to explain the retro-orbital or periorbital pain which usually precedes the onset of the ocular muscle palsy. Other authors have postulated compression of the third nerve between the origins of the posterior cerebral and superior cerebellar arteries. While it cannot be denied that these arteries may be distended during the migraine process, this theory does not correlate well with the situation of the headache and fails to explain the occasional abducens and trochlear nerve palsies.

The alternative hypothesis of segmental ischaemia of the oculomotor nerve resulting from migrainous angiospasm of the small branch of the internal carotid artery which supplies this nerve is difficult to accept. It would hardly account for the severe periorbital pain. Comparison with the clinical features of a diabetic oculomotor palsy, where an ischaemic aetiology is generally accepted, provides further evidence against segmental ischaemia as a cause of migrainous ophthalmoplegia. In diabetes, in contrast to migraine, pain is mild or absent and the pupil is not involved.

A mild unilateral ptosis occurs not infrequently in common or classic migraine; it is seen more often in cluster headache where it may be associated with miosis on the same side. Although this oculosympathetic paresis can persist for several days, it hardly qualifies for inclusion in the concept of complicated migraine.

Hemiplegic Migraine

The definition of this uncommon variant of migraine is here confined to attacks where hemiparesis, at times including the face, is a prominent feature.

This hemiparesis can occur only in a single attack, or it may recur and alternate from side to side. If we adhere to the concepts outlined earlier, hemiplegic migraine can be accepted as a form of complicated migraine only if the hemiparesis outlasts the headache. This has been the case in the majority of recorded cases.

There are two distinct forms of hemiplegic migraine; sporadic and familial. Both are rare, but reports of the sporadic form outnumber those of the familial variety. The majority of patients had also been subject to more simple attacks of migraine throughout their lives. Subjective sensations of heaviness or of loss of dexterity of an arm or hand, as well as a more definite paresis of a limb during the prodromal phase of an attack, were discussed in the description of classic migraine and will not be reiterated here. In the hemiplegic form of complicated migraine, just as in the ophthalmic or ophthalmoplegic forms, the physical disabilities outlast the headache and may persist for days or weeks.

The following case histories illustrate clinical features which justify a diagnosis of hemiplegic migraine.

A 60-year-old farmer was admitted to hospital in September, 1978. He had suffered from classic migraine since youth; most of the attacks were heralded by seeing spots before his right eye. The ensuing right frontal headache was accompanied by photophobia and nausea. At the age of 54 years an exceptionally severe right hemicrania was followed by a right hemiparesis including the face and by numbness of the right half of his body. His wife reported that he became mentally confused; he has no clear recollection of events during the next two weeks. He was admitted to a hospital in another city. The hemiparesis and numbness of the right side of his body recovered completely within two weeks. Six years later he again had a severe right hemicrania and temporarily lost vision in his right eye. At the height of the headache the right half of his body became numb, but this time he had no hemiparesis. He recovered from the headache and numbness within two days. His brother also suffered from migraine, but had never been hemiparetic. When this patient was admitted to our hospital some ten weeks after the last episode, examination showed no residual weakness or objective sensory impairment. Tendon and superficial reflexes were normal and symmetrical. He had a moderate hypertension with blood pressure readings ranging from 22/12.7kPa (165/95mm Hg) to 24/14.7kPa (180/110mm Hg). No bruits were heard over the carotid arteries. The results of electroencephalography, nuclear brain scan and computerized tomographic brain scan were normal, as were the results of chest X-ray examination, electrocardiography, blood count and serum chemistry, except for a mild elevation of cholesterol and triglyceride levels. Serological tests for syphilis were negative.

The diagnosis of complicated migraine in this patient was based on his history of classic migraine since youth and on the fact that the temporary right hemiparesis in 1972, as well as the numbness of the right side of his body in the same episode and again in 1978, were on the same side as his hemicrania. Radiological and imaging procedures had provided no evidence for a structural cerebral lesion.

The next case history describes a younger patient where clinical features suggested a diagnosis of hemiplegic migraine even in the absence of a previous history of vascular headache.

A truck driver, aged 31 years, was suddenly smitten with an excruciatingly severe occipital headache during sexual intercourse. He remained fully conscious and did not feel bilious. Within a few minutes he discovered that he could not see at all with his right eye. He tested his vision in each eye separately and was emphatic that he could see normally with the left eye, while the right eye was completely blind. He then noticed a paresis of his right arm and of the right side of his face and experienced paraesthesia which involved the right arm more than the right leg. Headache and loss of vision in the right eye recovered completely within 40 minutes, but the weakness and paraesthesia persisted. He had not previously been subject to migraine, but his father was known to have suffered from this malady. He was admitted to hospital in another city three days after these dramatic events when examination still showed a mild paresis and increased tendon reflexes in the right upper limb. He had no neck stiffness. A bruit was heard over the left subclavian artery, but blood pressures were normal and equal in the two arms. Routine laboratory investigations, including blood count, erythrocyte sedimentation rate, biochemical profile and X-ray examinations of his skull and chest, gave normal results; serological tests for syphilis were negative. The computerized tomographic (CT) brain scan gave entirely normal results. An arch aortogram, bilateral carotid arteriograms and selective left subclavian angiogram showed no abnormalities in the carotid circulation on both sides. A localized narrowing of the second part of the left subclavian artery, distal to the origin of the vertebral artery, was demonstrated. This was the cause of the bruit. The radiologist and a vascular surgeon interpreted this narrowing as due to external compression of the artery, possibly from a fibrous band and related to a past injury in which he had fractured the left clavicle. The mild paresis of the right arm recovered completely within a week. The CT brain scan was repeated after a few weeks and results were again normal. This patient was referred to me some ten months after this disturbing episode because he was very concerned about the possibility of a recurrence and had developed a variety of psychosomatic complaints. Apart from the left subclavian bruit, physical examination was unremarkable.

In this patient the diagnosis of hemiplegic migraine rests on the severity of the initial headache and on the transient loss of vision in the right eye alone; that is, on the same side as the weakness and paraesthesia. Although the cerebrospinal fluid had not been examined, the recovery from headache within 40 minutes and the absence of neck stiffness made a diagnosis of subarachnoid haemorrhage very unlikely.

The above two case histories were described in some detail because the possibility of hemiplegic migraine had hardly been considered by the physicians who saw the patients initially. In both cases, a diagnosis of occlusive stroke was mentioned and the patients remained apprehensive about their prognosis.

Although hemiparesis is rare in comparison with cortical visual and sensory disorders in complicated migraine, it is entirely reasonable to assume that the pathogenetic mechanism is identical; namely, constriction of distal small branches of the middle cerebral artery supplying the motor cortex or subcortical parts of the corticospinal tract. This assumption is supported by the alternating sides of hemiplegia and by the occasional observation of bilateral extensor plantar responses in patients where only one side was hemiplegic in an attack. Mild constriction of these vessels causes only oedema in the ischaemic area and clinical recovery occurs within a few hours or days. However, if the arterial spasm is sufficiently intense and prolonged, complete occlusion of the vessel and infarction of the brain may result, just as was shown to occur in the retina.

Dorfman et al. (1979) have recently documented cerebral infarction by serial computed cranial tomography and cerebral arteriography in four young adults with migraine. In one of these the infarct was shown to be of haemorrhagic type in the contrast-enhanced computerized tomographic (CT) brain scan. Occlusion of a small branch of the posterior cerebral artery was demonstrated in the arteriograms of only one of their patients, while no major arterial occlusions were seen in the films from the other three patients. However, serial CT scans showed unequivocal signs of cerebral infarction. Exhaustive laboratory investigations in two of these patients excluded all the usually accepted risk factors for cerebral infarction; in three patients, the infarct occurred in the territory involved in previous uncomplicated attacks of migraine. Two patients were left with lasting neurological deficits. The work of Dorfman et al. confirms that migraine is not always a benign disease. The following case history supports this contention.

A 43-year-old left-handed German-born woman had suffered from classic migraine for 20 years. The attacks were infrequent, occurring from two to four times a year, during the first 15 years, but then their frequency increased to one to four each month. A visual aura of shimmering lights and serrated lines (in both visual fields) and bilateral tunnel vision lasting some 20 minutes preceded the headache which was always confined to the right frontal region; it was associated with photophobia and vomiting. She was aware of a family history of migraine only in a maternal aunt and cousin.

In June, 1978, she had three severe attacks over a period of three days. Immediately after the third attack she abruptly developed an expressive non-fluent dysphasia, as well as difficulty with writing and mathematical calculations. A few hours later a left hemiparesis appeared, involving the arm more than the leg. She was admitted to hospital in another city. Electroencephalography (EEG) showed focal slow activity from the right frontal area and the computerized tomographic (CT) brain scan, with and without contrast infusion, demonstrated a haemorrhagic infarct, surrounded by oedema, in the right frontoparietal region. Extensive investigations failed to reveal any risk factors for cerebral vascular disease.

The left hemiparesis had disappeared within three weeks, but an expressive dysphasia was still evident when I examined this lady three months after her migrainous cerebral infarction. She was then normally fluent in her native German, but was still hesitant finding words in English which she had spoken fluently before the onset of her dysphasia. There was no residual weakness of her left limbs; tendon and superficial reflexes were normal and symmetrical. A progress CT brain scan in September, 1978, showed only a small area of decreased density, consistent with an old infarct, in the right parietal region. This did not enhance with contrast. Subsequently, she continued to have attacks of predominantly right frontal migraine, mainly in association with menstruation which were not complicated by dysphasia or hemiparesis. In May, 1979, she had a single Jacksonian epileptic seizure; convulsive movements began in her left arm and spread to the face and leg before she lost consciousness. An EEG showed sharply contoured slow waves from the right frontal region, indicating that this seizure had probably arisen from the area of infarction. She was treated with anticonvulsant drugs and reported no further seizures when reviewed six months later.

In this case, as in those reported by Dorfman *et al.* (1979), the relationship of cerebral infarction to migraine is beyond reasonable doubt. With the increasing use of computerized tomographic brain scanning, it is likely that many more similar cases will be reported during the next few years.

Familial hemiplegic migraine has several features which distinguish it from the sporadic (non-familial) variety described above. During the past 70 years only a few reports in the literature have devoted attention to this rare condition. Over two to four generations, several members of a family may be afflicted; transmission is autosomal dominant. Hemiplegia tends to recur at varying intervals. In some families it involved the same side in all members; in others, as well as in some individual patients, it alternated from side to side. The onset of hemiplegia can be abrupt and complete restoration of normal motor power within days or weeks is the rule. Hemicrania was ipsilateral to the hemiplegia in about one-third of cases reported in detail (Bradshaw and Parsons, 1965). Dysphasia, as well as visual and sensory disorders, occurred either in association with hemiparesis or separately in a proportion of cases. As a preceding history of attacks of typical migraine was reported by most patients, there is little justification for the view that familial hemiplegic migraine differs from other types of migraine from a nosological point of view. However, it is intriguing to speculate what exactly is inherited over several generations of a family to produce an episodic hemiplegia which can involve the same limbs in all affected members and yet exhibits no signs of a structural cerebral lesion.

In several of the cases of familial hemiplegic migraine cited in the literature, attacks of hemiparesis were followed by severe and initially transient intellectual

disorders (dysphrenic migraine) and by drowsiness and disturbances of consciousness of varying degrees of severity (Symonds, 1951; Blau and Whitty, 1955;
Bradshaw and Parsons, 1965). I had the good fortune to work in Sir Charles
Symonds' ward at the National Hospital for Nervous Diseases, Queen Square,
London, when one of these patients was admitted. His story was described in
some detail in a paper on "Migrainous Variants" by Symonds in 1951. The
patient, a male aged 48 years at the time of his admission to the National Hospital, had suffered from classic migraine since childhood. The attacks occurred
from one to three times a year and began with a gradual loss of vision, numbness
and weakness on one side, followed by headache, vomiting and drowsiness. He
usually recovered from the right sided attacks within 48 hours, but, if the hemiparesis involved the left side, he passed into a state of coma. Hemiparesis and
coma persisted for four to five days. He remained confused for a further three
to four days. His father had suffered from exactly similar attacks since childhood
and at the age of 62 years was admitted to a psychiatric hospital where he died
four years later. The patient recalled that his paternal grandfather had also been
subject to similar attacks. During one of this man's previous hospital admissions,
a complete left homonymous hemianopia, impairment of cutaneous and deep
sensibility on the left side, as well as a dense left hemiplegia with appropriate
changes in the tendon and superficial reflexes, were recorded. The cerebrospinal
fluid was examined during several admissions and once contained 185 poly-
morphonuclear neutrophils/mm^3, but there were no abnormal chemical constituents. Three days later the number of neutrophils had fallen to 5/mm^3. An air
encephalogram, performed a few days later, showed no abnormality. When he
was admitted to the National Hospital on the third day of an attack in 1950, he
was drowsy and confused and again had a complete left homonymous hemianopia, dense left hemiplegia and left hemihypaesthesia. The cerebrospinal fluid
contained 3 neutrophils/mm^3; the chemical constituents of the fluid were in the
normal range. A right carotid arteriogram showed no abnormality, but in the
electroencephalogram (EEG) the alpha activity from the right hemisphere was
suppressed and slow delta frequencies were recorded from the right frontal and
parietal regions, in addition to some bilateral slow activity. The EEG gradually
returned to normal within eight days, coincident with complete clinical recovery.

Symonds (1951) suggests that his detailed observations of this remarkable
case are consistent with the hypothesis of recurrent and widespread, though predominantly unilateral, vascular spasm as a cause of the attacks. This accounts
for the complete clinical recovery from each episode, for the gross abnormalities
in the EEG at the height of an attack, and for the subsequent improvement in
the brain's electrical activity, simultaneous with the disappearance of abnormal
clinical signs. The neutrophil pleocytosis demonstrated in the cerebrospinal fluid
during three of this patient's attacks could be attributed to small cerebral infarctions. Symonds goes on to propose that such repeated small infarctions may
have a cumulative effect, causing structural brain damage which contributed to
the progressive dementia of the patient's father. What a pity that computerized
brain scanning was not available at that time to support this assumption.

Dysphrenic Migraine

The term "dysphrenic" refers to states of confusion, defects of memory and
impairment of intellectual functions which may occur during the course of a

migraine attack. In complicated migraine this loss of mental alacrity goes beyond the slight difficulties in concentration, attention and organization of ideas which many patients experience either during the premonitory or headache phase of common or classic migraine. The spectrum of mental disorders ranges from confusion, disorientation, amnesia and agitation to hallucinations, phobias, depression, mania and other psychotic states. Many of the most severe disorders of mood and behaviour were reported in the literature before 1930. In some patients, personality traits and psychotic behaviour patterns unrelated to their migraine attacks leave us in some doubt as to whether the mental aberrations were an integral part of their migraine syndrome. However, there is a clear analogy between the various mental aberrations and the visual and neurological disorders in migraine which we have described earlier: they are transient; they can, at times, occur without headache; they may be coincident with visual or focal cerebral symptoms; and, in complicated migraine, they may persist for prolonged periods.

Dysphrenic migraine is uncommon. Therefore, the diagnosis is easily missed and depends largely on a detailed history. I had the opportunity to follow the progress of such a patient over a period of 17 years.

A boy of 13 years was admitted to hospital in 1963 for investigation of a severe right hemicrania accompanied by vomiting and marked mental confusion. He became very drowsy within a few hours, but could still be aroused. He had no neck stiffness, nor were any abnormal neurological signs present. A diagnosis of viral encephalitis was suspected, but the cerebrospinal fluid contained no excess of cells nor any abnormal chemical constituents. The electroencephalogram showed an excess of bilateral slow activity, both in the delta and theta range. The headache abated and he became mentally alert within three days. At that time, the electroencephalographic results returned to normal. His father and paternal grandmother suffered from migraine.

Over the next 17 years, he had only four or five episodes of severe headache and photophobia; one of these was associated with mental confusion lasting a few hours and another with paraesthesia of his right limbs. In August, 1980, he felt dizzy and complained of bilateral blurring of vision which persisted for 30 minutes. He attempted to drive home, but was seen to drive erratically and progressively slower. Eventually, he drove the car off the road and towards a tree, but sustained no injury. Friends found him stuporous and he was taken to hospital. He responded to pain, but not to vocal stimuli. Within an hour of admission he became restless and irritable and vomited. He was intensely photophobic and did not permit examination of his optic fundi. He had no neck stiffness; neurological and general examinations were unremarkable. The cerebrospinal fluid contained no cells and normal amounts of protein and glucose. On the next day he was still drowsy and photophobic, but was able to co-operate in the performance of a full neurological examination. The electroencephalogram then showed episodic delta frequencies of high amplitude from both frontal regions, as well as theta activity from the left temporo-occipital area, enhanced by hyperventilation. Results of computerized tomographic brain scan were normal.

His headache subsided and he became normally alert over the next 48 hours, but he had no recollection of his car running off the road, of his admission to hospital or of the events during his first 30 hours in hospital. A progress EEG, obtained some eight weeks later, did not show any bifrontal or left temporo-occipital slow activity; the tracing was entirely normal.

The normal results from computerized tomographic brain scan in 1980 excluded a structural cerebral lesion, while the grossly abnormal findings in the electroencephalograms performed during his stupor, irritability and amnesia (with subsequent return to normal tracings) both in 1963 and 1980 suggested a transient disorder of cerebral function. Severe headache, vomiting and photophobia and the few intervening episodes of migraine established that this disorder had a migrainous aetiology.

We have already referred to transient dysphrenic symptoms recorded during attacks of familial hemiplegic migraine. Any combination of visual, sensory or mental disorders can occur in individual attacks during the lifespan of a person with complicated migraine. The following case history describes such a patient's progress over a period of 13 years.

An eight-year-old boy was first admitted to hospital in 1967. Attacks of classic migraine began when he was only three years old and gradually increased in frequency from four to 10-12 a year. He first complained of pain in the left supraorbital region; then vision in his left eye became dimmed so that he could hardly see. In some attacks, his level of awareness was reduced, some adversion of his head to the left was noted and his limbs "shivered" a little. Headache and vomiting continued for about two hours, after which he fell asleep. On waking he was always perfectly well. He had a family history of migraine on the maternal side and of post-traumatic epilepsy in one of his paternal relatives.

In February, 1967, one of these attacks was followed by loss of consciousness for about two hours. Breathing was stertorous and restless movements of his arms, rather than epileptiform convulsions, were noted. On arrival at the hospital, he had regained his senses, but was drowsy. Neurological examination was unrewarding. The tracing of the first electroencephalogram (EEG), recorded soon after his admission, was disorganized, with continuous bilateral slow activity and focal slow and sharply contoured complexes from the right mid-temporal area. Two days later, the basic organization of the EEG tracing improved markedly, but focal abnormalities from the right temporal area remained. The cerebrospinal fluid contained three monocytes and normal chemical constituents. The right carotid angiogram and a pneumoencephalogram were entirely normal.

One month later, he vomited at school, became dazed and developed focal seizures involving the left limbs. They lasted about 90 seconds and then recurred every 10 minutes over a period of two hours. He was just rousable, but on the following day he was again perfectly well. He was then treated with phenytoin and primidone. Focal slow activity from the right posterior temporal region persisted in the results of progress EEGs recorded over the next four years; then the EEG focus switched to the left temporo-occipital area. During the second half of 1973 he had about six mild generalized convulsive seizures, usually associated with a febrile illness. During the following two years no further seizures occurred, but he reported four episodes of partial or complete loss of vision in the left eye, each lasting two to five minutes. Only one of these was followed by headache. Five years later, early in 1980, he reported episodes of abrupt loss of vision in the temporal field of the left eye, which recovered after five to seven minutes. The visual loss was followed immediately by an expressive dysphasia which also persisted for only a few minutes. He could always understand what was said to him and was able to nod in reply. Some 10 to 15 minutes later he experienced a dull left frontal headache and nausea. These attacks had occurred at an average of about one a month. The EEG tracing no longer showed any focal or diffuse slow activity and was normal. A computerized tomographic brain scan, with and without contrast, showed no abnormality.

The last two case histories show that not only mental aberrations, but also prolonged episodes of coma, as well as partial or generalized seizures can occur during attacks of complicated migraine. These alarming events are of such magnitude that the diagnosis of migraine may not immediately come to mind. The "dysphrenic" symptoms can be attributed to ischaemia of the frontal or temporal lobes and there is no reason why these parts of the brain should be spared in the vasoconstrictive, ischaemic phase of a migraine attack, even though the occipital (visual disorders) and parietal (sensory symptoms) lobes are more frequently affected.

The diverse and protean clinical manifestations of classic or complicated migraine provide the physician with a unique opportunity to witness and study the entire spectrum of cerebral dysfunction. A single concept of focal or multifocal cerebral or retinal ischaemia serves to explain all symptoms with the exception of the ocular palsies in ophthalmoplegic migraine which appear to result from nerve compression by distended arteries. Mild ischaemia may cause symptoms of neuronal excitation, while a more severe degree of reduced perfusion temporarily inhibits neuronal function. The nature and severity of focal symptoms can change from attack to attack. The transient nature, and the tendency for complete recovery, of these symptoms in the overwhelming majority of cases can best be explained on a vascular basis. Although experimental observations have suggested that vasoconstriction may be diffuse and bilateral, it appears to vary in degree in different areas of the brain. Slight intracranial vasoconstriction causes mild ischaemia and some oedema of the affected brain tissue, and these produce the very brief focal disturbances observed during the aura of an attack of classic migraine. The severity and duration of symptoms is proportional to the degree and duration of vasoconstriction. If this is frequently repeated and severe, infarction will result and symptoms may then persist for prolonged periods and may even become permanent. Recurrent ischaemia or infarction in the same or adjoining regions of the brain can have a cumulative effect and produce progressive disorders of intellect or of visual, sensory or motor function. Gross, but temporary abnormalities in the EEG tracings and, less often, in the results of computerized tomographic brain scans, confirm the contention that the disorder of structure and function of parts of the brain in migraine is transient.

We have provided clinical evidence that any of the branches of the carotid or vertebral arteries can be involved, excepting only those which supply the cerebellum. As yet, we have no explanation why the cerebellum should be spared in migraine, nor do we know why the same arterial territory may be constricted in each attack in a small proportion of patients. The hereditary form of hemiplegic migraine is the most challenging reminder of our ignorance of some fundamental events in the pathogenesis of migraine. We can only assume that there is not only a generalized abnormal vascular reactivity, but also a more profound disorder restricted to small segments of the arterial tree. This could be attributed to an increased regional concentration of vasoactive amines, which facilitate or maintain excessive vasoconstriction in the repeatedly involved vascular territory. As an alternative hypothesis, it is possible that small areas of brain, cortical or subcortical, which were rendered ischaemic in previous attacks, become more susceptible to even a minor degreee of vasoconstriction, no greater than that which simultaneously involves other parts of the brain. This means that the threshold of stimulation or inhibition of these areas has been reduced and that similar focal symptoms will, therefore, appear in each attack.

It was mentioned during the discussion of classic and complicated migraine that the excessive vasoconstriction extends to the terminal branches of both the carotid and basilar tree. Branches of the retinal arteries are more often involved than any other vessels, while the less common episodes of vertigo, at least in a proportion of cases, implicate the labyrinthine end arteries. The widely held view that arterial distension *must* follow after constriction is no longer tenable. Just as distension of extracranial vessels occurs in common migraine without symptoms indicative of intracranial vasoconstriction, so focal visual or neurological disturbances, resulting from such constriction, can occur in classic migraine without headache. This implies that constriction of intracranial vessels may be an entirely separate event from the painful dilation of extracranial arteries. Therefore, migrainous angiospastic symptoms can occur without ensuing headache.

Migraine Without Headache

In the description of classic migraine we have mentioned that some patients may, at times, experience only the visual, sensory or labyrinthine symptoms of their aura without the later appearance of the expected headache. In these cases the diagnosis of migraine presents no difficulty. However, there are a few people who have visual hallucinations or scotomata identical to those usually seen in migraine, but who had never suffered from migraine or other forms of headache. The visual disorders may be bilateral or may alternate from side to side. They rarely last longer than 20 minutes, and can be distinguished from episodes of amaurosis fugax or retinal vascular lesions only by obtaining a careful history and full ophthalmoscopic examination.

The following two case histories were obtained from reliable and intelligent patients.

A psychiatrist, aged 58 years, described several transient episodes of visual disorder over a period of nine months. He suddenly saw a serrated crescent of shimmering lights which gradually expanded from the centre towards the periphery of the visual field of both eyes. In most attacks, this crescent was associated with a bilateral partial scotoma near the centre of his visual field. The scintillating crescents persisted when his eyes were shut; each episode lasted for periods of from 20 to 35 minutes. There was no pain in his eyes or head during or after the visual symptoms. He had never suffered from migraine in the past and no family history of this disorder was known. No abnormality was found on neurological or ophthalmological examination. No bruits were heard in the neck or over the orbits. Blood pressure was 16.3kPa (122mm Hg) systolic and 10.9kPa (82mm Hg) diastolic. Serum chemistry, including measurement of fasting glucose, cholesterol and triglyceride levels, was normal.

The second history of similar symptoms concerns a 41-year-old airline pilot whose occupation was handicapped by unpredictable, though infrequent, disturbances of vision:

Over a period of ten years this patient had about eight attacks which followed a similar pattern. None was provoked by any specific events in his environment and none had occurred while he was flying. He first saw a bright dot in the centre of his visual field; this then assumed jagged edges and slowly moved towards the periphery of the visual field. While the shimmering dot was in the centre of his field of vision he could not see distinctly, but his vision returned to normal as it moved towards the periphery. He was not certain if one or both eyes were affected. The visual disorder continued for about five minutes with the exception of one attack where it lasted for just over an hour. There was no ensuing headache, but he usually felt slightly bilious just after his sight returned to normal. He had never suffered from migraine or other headache in the past. No information about his family history could be obtained. Neurological and ophthalmological examination showed no abnormality. Results of a computerized tomographic brain scan and a nuclear brain scan were normal.

In each of the above two patients, a diagnosis of migraine would be accepted without question if at least some of the visual symptoms had been followed by headache, or if a past history of vascular headache of migraine type had been obtained. It may be argued that migrainous retinal angiospasm can hardly be postulated in the complete absence of headache. This argument is weakened by the common occurrence of identical symptoms during the aura of a typical attack of classic migraine and, at times, without the expected headache in the same patient. We have already pointed out that constriction of cerebral or retinal arteries may occur quite independently of later dilation of extracranial vessels.

Further evidence for this concept is provided by the occurrence of recurrent, brief episodes of vertigo in middle aged persons who had suffered from common or classic migraine during their youth. Symonds (1951) had noted vertiginous attacks in nearly 10% of 500 cases of migraine and assumed that they were due to localized spasm of labyrinthine arteries. He observed that the duration of vertigo was much shorter than the visual or sensory symptoms of the migraine aura, usually lasting only one or two minutes, but occasionally continuing for up to 20 minutes. The absence of deafness and aural discomfort distinguishes this angiospastic labyrinthine vertigo from Meniere's syndrome.

I have seen several women with a history of migraine over many years, which would abate at the time of the menopause when brief episodes of vertigo without headache appeared in place of the previous migraine.

A doctor's secretary, aged 49 years, had suffered from common migraine, often associated with menstruation, since youth. The frequency and severity of her attacks had declined in recent years. After the age of 47 years she began to complain of recurrent episodes of rotational vertigo, non-directional ataxia and nausea. Each attack lasted from 10 to 15 minutes and none was associated with headache. The frequency of attacks had gradually increased from one a month to four to six a month. Some attacks always occurred during the menses. She first experienced a pressure sensation in her head. A few seconds later her environment seemed to spin and move around her. She was so unsteady that she preferred to lie down immediately and shut her eyes. There was no feeling of fullness in her ears, but on a few occasions she had a mild bilateral tinnitus. No diplopia or other symptoms of brain stem dysfunction were ever noted. Her mother, sister and two daughters also suffered from migraine. The findings on neurological and otological examination were unrewarding. Audiography confirmed that the patient had normal hearing, but the caloric tests revealed a slightly reduced vestibular response on the right side.

A second case of migrainous vertigo is described because this patient also had hypertension and a diagnosis of transient vertebrobasilar ischaemia had been suspected.

A 67-year-old widow had suffered from attacks of common migraine since childhood; the headaches were severe, either unilateral or generalized and had been associated with photophobia and vomiting. They occurred at the time of menstruation and ceased at the menopause. When she was 65 years old, she began to suffer from short episodes of rotational vertigo. These continued intermittently over a period of six weeks, then stopped and recurred 18 months later. Vertigo usually appeared soon after waking in the morning and lasted for only a few minutes. It appeared to her that objects were rocking or spinning around her. This sensation was immediately aggravated by moving her head. If she tried to walk, she veered towards the left. She perspired and felt bilious, but did not vomit. Her hearing was normal and she had no tinnitus. The brief episodes of vertigo were not followed by headache, but she felt exhausted and preferred to rest for about an hour. She had never experienced diplopia or any neurological symptoms suggesting brain stem ischaemia. No abnormality was found on neurological or otological examination. However, she had asymptomatic hypertension and a hypertensive retinopathy.

It is of some interest that migrainous angiospasm without headache involves mainly vision and balance. The visual symptoms described by most patients favour ischaemia of the retina rather than of the visual cortex, while the aggravation of vertigo by head movement and the occasional abnormal caloric responses implicate the labyrinths rather than the central vestibular connections.

Although some migraineurs report transient sensory, motor, speech and even mental disorders without headache, the retinae and labyrinths are much more often affected. As the retinal arteries are terminal branches of the internal carotid and the labyrinthine arteries are terminal branches of the basilar artery, it is suggested that these small vessels are more susceptible to migrainous vasoconstriction.

If these visual or labyrinthine disorders occcur without headache, the diagnosis of migraine may not be initally considered. The association of scintillating, spreading crescents with transient central scotomata is quite different from the symptoms noted by patients with amaurosis fugax or various retinal vascular lesions and the physician who has seen such patients will have no difficulty in arriving at the correct diagnosis. Migrainous angiospastic vertigo is relatively uncommon. The preservation of normal hearing, with minimal or no tinnitus, and the brevity of attacks, distinguish this disorder from Meniere's syndrome. Although vertigo and ataxia may initially be the only symptoms of basilar ischaemia, the frequency and short duration of attacks, and a past history of migraine, should guide the physician towards a diagnosis of migrainous vertigo and avoid the performance of invasive or expensive investigations.

Lower Half Headache

The Ad Hoc Committee on Classification of Headache of the National Institute of Neurological Diseases and Blindness (1962) defined lower half headache as a pain of possibly vascular mechanism, centred primarily in the lower face. It is an uncommon condition, not well defined and, therefore, easily confused with some "atypical" facial neuralgias.

A diagnosis of lower half headache should be considered in persons who are also subject to more conventional forms of migraine and when the episodes of facial pain are prolonged and can reasonably be attributed to distension of branches of the external carotid artery. The pain often starts near the nose, then spreads to the cheek and ear; it may radiate down as far as the neck. Attacks usually last for a few hours, but may last days. The diagnosis of a migrainous aetiology is suggested by the concurrence of photophobia, nausea and vomiting.

The characteristic clinical features of lower half headache are described in the following two case histories.

A 48-year-old housewife was referred for treatment of trigeminal neuralgia which had not responded to carbamazepine. She had suffered from common migraine since she was 19 years old. During the last two years, she had suffered attacks of severe pain confined to the lower half of the face at irregular intervals. She might have attacks on eight successive days and then enjoy six weeks of freedom. The pain usually began near the tip of her nose and then radiated into both cheeks, towards her ears, down into the lower jaws and, at times, into the neck. Though usually bilateral, it had also involved the right or left side separately. The attacks lasted for an average of about nine hours; on several occasions, facial pain occurred simultaneously with her migrainous headaches and was then associated with photophobia and nausea. She had not recognized any triggers which evoked the facial pain. Some of her sisters suffered from migraine. No abnormalities were found on neurological examination, and there were no signs of temporomandibular joint dysfunction.

The long duration and bilateral situation of this woman's pain, as well as the absence of the usual triggers, made a diagnosis of trigeminal neuralgia untenable, while the past history and occasional concurrence with migraine clearly indicated that she suffered from a vascular type of facial neuralgia.

Another patient had no definite history of migraine, but the diagnosis of lower half headache was suggested by intense photophobia and nausea during each attack.

A woman aged 33 years with a family history of migraine in one of her sisters had fairly stereotyped attacks of facial pain for two years. In the first year, only four or five attacks occurred, but then their frequency increased to an average of three per month. The pain began at any time of the day or night and persisted for about six hours. It started in the right suboccipital region and rapidly spread around the right ear into the right middle face. The pain was so intense that she was forced to retire to bed; it was always accompanied by a feeling of pressure in the right eye and by marked photophobia and nausea. Neurological examination was unremarkable and movements of the cervical spine were free and painless in all directions. Propranolol failed to reduce the frequency of her attacks, but a compound preparation containing ergotamine provided relief within one to two hours. She refused to try methysergide because of its potential side effects.

Although lower half headache is uncommon, it is important to recognize it because it often responds to treatment for migraine. It differs from cluster headache where the attacks occur in bouts and the pain is felt mainly in the forehead and around the eye. In general, each attack of cluster headache is also much shorter than the duration of pain in lower half headache. It is not difficult to distinguish it from trigeminal neuralgia as the paroxysms of pain in tic douloureux are usually triggered by chewing, talking, or touching the face. They follow the distribution of one or more branches of the trigeminal nerve and generally last for only a few minutes, though they may recur at frequent intervals. Treatment with carbamazepine, which is often temporarily effective in trigeminal neuralgia, fails in lower half headache. Pain caused by temporomandibular joint dysfunction involves an area of the face similar to lower half headache, but is usually evoked by chewing or talking. Generally, the attacks of pain last less than an hour, the temporomandibular joints may be tender to pressure and an irregularity of the bite may be noted. The absence of photophobia and nausea and the lack of a past or concurrent history of migraine would also favour a diagnosis of temporomandibular joint dysfunction (Costen's syndrome). In the various forms of atypical facial neuralgia, many of which are psychogenic, pain is persistent and continuous for months or years. It is often bilateral, and not associated with photophobia, nausea or headache.

It is unfortunate that many patients with lower half headache are referred to the neurologist only after prolonged and unsuccessful treatment from dental and medical practitioners. This treatment has even included injection of alcohol into branches of the trigeminal nerve.

Cluster Headache

Though relatively uncommon, cluster headache is an important variant of vascular headache because of the extreme severity of pain. The condition responds well to treatment. Isolated cases were described for over a century and many were confused with other forms of poorly defined neuralgias in the head and face. Various descriptive terms and eponyms, such as red migraine, erythroprosopalgia, erythromelalgia of the head, sphenopalatine neuralgia and vidian neuralgia, were proposed and added to the nosological confusion. Harris (1926) was the first to propose a relationship of the syndrome to migraine and described its essential features under the heading "Periodic Migrainous Neuralgia". Ten years later (Harris, 1936), he used the term "ciliary neuralgia" when the pain was felt mainly in or behind the eye. The essential characteristic of the headache to occur in bouts or clusters was emphasized by Kunkle *et al.* (1952), who introduced the name cluster headache. This has since gained wide acceptance.

As there are both similarities to and differences from other variants of migraine, some authors have questioned whether cluster headache should be included in the concept of migraine or regarded as an entirely distinct variety of headache. It is certainly a vascular type of headache, though almost invariably confined to the extracranial vessels, and the similarities to migraine may be greater than the differences. Therefore, cluster headache was included under the heading of "vascular headache of migraine type" by the Ad Hoc Committee on Classification of Headache in 1962.

No reliable surveys of the prevalence of cluster headache are available. A minimal prevalence of 4.5 cases per 100 000 of population was suggested by Sutherland and Eadie (1972). This is probably an underestimate because most neurologists agree that the diagnosis is frequently missed. In a series of 28 patients, Balla and Walton (1964) found only one who had been correctly diagnosed at the time of referral; they also noted that the average delay in diagnosis was 6.5 years after the first attack.

In contrast to the female preponderance of common and classic migraine, cluster headache occurs predominantly in males in a ratio of about 4:1. The disease rarely begins in the first two decades of life; the common age of onset is between 20 and 50 years with a mean of 30 to 35 years. The clusters then continue for many years, but tend to diminish after the age of 60. A family history of cluster headache is very rare and occurs in less than 1% of cases. However, a positive family history of other forms of migraine can be obtained from 5% to 35% of patients with cluster headache. This is much lower than the 50% to 75% incidence of a positive family history in common or classic migraine, but it is higher than figures available for the non-migrainous population. A stronger point in favour of a link between migraine and cluster headache is a personal history of common or classic migraine either before the first cluster or in the often long intervals between clusters in some 12% to 25% of patients. In contrast with common migraine, no specific environmental triggers for cluster headache can be elicited from the majority of patients. In some subjects, the attacks occurred mainly during spring; others were able to relate some clusters to emotional stress, but readily admitted that they had experienced many similar stress situations without an attack. In some 10% of cases reported in the literature, alcohol precipitated a cluster or, more often, elicited a paroxysm during a cluster.

Pathophysiology

There is a consensus that localized extracranial vasodilation in the periorbital region contributes to the pain of cluster headache. This is supported by the almost invariable conjunctival congestion, the less common flushing of the face and the relief obtained from vasoconstrictor drugs. In contrast to migraine, it is said that the ophthalmic arteries as well as the small arterioles and capillaries of the scalp and face are dilated, in addition to the dilation of the extracranial arteries. This dilation is strictly unilateral; in migraine it is usually bilateral and only more marked on the side of the headache. No explanation has so far been offered why the pain of cluster headache is much more agonizing than pain in other forms of migraine. The occurrence of Horner's syndrome on the side of pain, and, perhaps, the nasal stuffiness and congestion on the same side, are indicative of cervical sympathetic paralysis. Although this may be secondary to severe dilation of the internal carotid artery below the siphon, the alternate possibility that this localized sympathetic paralysis is a primary event in the pathogenesis of cluster headache cannot be entirely dismissed. Symptoms of intracranial vasoconstriction are usually lacking; only isolated cases were described where migrainous visual prodromata appeared. Usually, they occurred in the intervals between paroxysms of cluster headache and were followed by symptoms of more conventional migraine.

Biochemistry

It was mentioned in Chapter 3 that plasma serotonin levels fall significantly during migraine headache (p25) and that the mean blood levels of histamine do not rise before, during or after an attack of migraine (p26). These observations do not apply to cluster headache and this is one of the reasons why its relationship to migraine has been doubted. In cluster headache, plasma levels of serotonin do not fall; they show no consistent pattern of change before, during or after the paroxysm of pain. On the other hand, levels of whole blood histamine rise significantly during the attack in comparison with headache-free periods (Anthony and Lance, 1971). Recent experimental studies in monkeys have shown that histamine H_1 and H_2 receptors subserve vasodilation in the internal carotid circulation, while only H_2 receptors are present in external carotid vessels. However, H_1 or H_2 blockade with appropriate drugs is only partly effective in preventing attacks of cluster headache in humans (Anthony, Lance and Lord, 1978). It is also of interest that the administration of nitroglycerine will almost invariably precipitate an attack during a bout of cluster headache, but has no effect in other forms of migraine. The pharmacological mechanisms for this action of nitroglycerine are not understood.

Although an injection of histamine produces pain, it is not known whether endogenous histamine is capable of doing the same. It is claimed that histamine release is associated with a simultaneous acceleration of histamine formation in various tissues — the newly formed histamine will then act within the cells and tissues of its origin. Anthony (1972b) proposed the hypothesis that, in cluster headache, an unknown stimulus sets off the release of stored histamine. This can occur rapidly and cause the dilation of small arteries, arterioles and capillaries. The released histamine is rapidly metabolized — its concentration in the blood falls, the distended blood vessels regain their tone and the clinical attack ends. Antihistamine drugs, which have no effect in the treatment of cluster headache, can act only on circulating histamine and not on the amine formed and active at tissue level. Corticosteroids inhibit histamine formation by reducing the activity of the enzyme histidine decarboxylase and are often effective in the prevention of cluster headaches. While this hypothesis would account for some of the clinical features of cluster headache, it fails to explain the predominant periorbital and supraorbital situation of the pain, its invariable recurrence on the same side during a single bout, and the "clockwork" regularity with which some of the paroxysms recur. Horton, who devoted many years to the study of periodic migrainous neuralgia, was convinced of the importance of histamine in its aetiology and proposed the term "histaminic cephalgia" (Horton, 1941, 1956). Initially, he appeared to be unaware of the occurrence of these headaches in bouts which terminated spontaneously and he erroneously claimed success from treatment with histamine desensitization. The clinical features of Horton's patients leave no doubt that they were suffering from what is now known as cluster headache. Some authors have paid tribute to his work by calling the disease "Horton's syndrome".

Clinical Features

Cluster headache has characteristic clinical features which make it possible for the physician who is aware of the condition to make a confident diagnosis with only a few exceptions. The features are as follows.

1.The paroxysms of pain occur in bouts or clusters. The average duration of a cluster ranges from two to ten weeks and the majority are shorter than four weeks. In a small proportion of patients, the paroxysmal attacks continue for months or even years. This rare variant, which can no longer be strictly called "cluster" headache, will be described later as it may be amenable to a specific form of treatment.

2. Initially, the clusters may occur during the same season each year, but the seasonal incidence tends to change or disappear later in the course of the disease. Clusters usually recur over many years and a duration of the illness exceeding 30 years has been reported (Friedman and Mikropoulos, 1958).

3. Intervals of complete freedom from headache range from three months to 25 years. In about 40% of patients, remissions last for less than 12 months.

4. During an individual cluster, an average of one to three paroxysms of pain occur during a 24-hour period, though patients may have up to six attacks each day. Both the frequency and periodicity of attacks tend to diminish as the cluster approaches its natural termination.

5. About two-thirds of the attacks occur during the night, often between midnight and 3am. At times, the pain will recur with clockwork regularity at precisely the same hour each night or day. This is one of the unique, fascinating and puzzling characteristics of this disease; in the future it may be explained in relation to circadian rhythms. In addition to these "clockwork" attacks, others may occur at random. In some patients, or in different clusters in the same person, there is no regularity in the timing of attacks; in many, the initial regular periodicity disappears in the later stages of a single cluster.

6. The duration of pain ranges from 10 minutes to several hours with an average of from 30 to 120 minutes. In about 60% of attacks the pain lasts for less than two hours and in 78% for less than three hours (Sutherland and Eadie, 1972).

7. The pain is almost invariably unilateral and remains on the same side in a single cluster. In later clusters it may change to the other side, though this is uncommon. In about four-fifths of patients the pain is felt in, behind and above the eye. Often it radiates towards the temple; less often, into the same side of the face and to the ear; more rarely, it extends to the occiput or even into the neck.

8. The onset of pain is rapid and progresses within minutes to its maximum severity. It is incapacitating, agonizing and terrifying in its intensity and is often described as throbbing, boring or burning. Many patients cannot remain still and feel compelled to move about and some will even bang their head on a wall in a vain effort to get relief. Some have contemplated suicide but, to the writer's knowledge, this was never carried out. The paroxysm abates more gradually than it started, but relief is usually complete.

9. Conjunctival congestion and lacrimation on the side of pain characterize most attacks; a feeling of blockage or stuffiness of the ipsilateral nostril, often associated with a clear or watery nasal discharge, occurs with a slightly lower frequency. Some patients report excessive perspiration of the ipsilateral eyebrow and cheek. These symptoms indicate parasympathetic overactivity, which may possibly be "liberated" by sympathetic paralysis.

10. Ipsilateral Horner's syndrome, caused by sympathetic paralysis, was reported in from 5% to 20% of attacks. At times, only a ptosis is mentioned, but in at least some of these patients the size of the pupils may not have been critically observed in a mirror or by witnesses to the attack. Occasional swelling of the affected side of the face, or redness of the ear and face, reflect the cutaneous vasodilation and motivated the early descriptive terms of "red migraine" and "erythromelalgia of the head".

11. Photophobia is unusual in comparison with migraine and is reported by no more than 10% to 30% of patients. The absence of photophobia in spite of marked congestion of the conjunctiva is of some interest as it provides evidence against the theory that congestion of conjunctival vessels is an important cause of photophobia. Nausea and vomiting, which occur so frequently with attacks of migraine are rare in cluster headache and are reported in less than 25% of attacks.

12. Apart from the occasional Horner's syndrome, neurological examination during an attack shows no abnormality. Electroencephalograms performed during a cluster, though not during an actual paroxysm of pain, were either normal or showed only non-specific bilateral slow activity. If a person suffering from cluster headache develops hypertension, the frequency, duration and severity of the attacks do not change.

No lasting complications of cluster headache have been reported. There are a few recorded instances of permanent Horner's syndrome and isolated cases of addiction to strong analgesic drugs. There have been reports of toxic effects from the prolonged use of large doses of ergotamines.

Symonds (1956a) provided the most complete, critical and erudite account of the condition up to that date. He described each of the clinical features which are now accepted as diagnostic criteria and illustrated them with case histories. Although he referred to the headings of "periodic migrainous neuralgia" and "cluster headache", and agrees that there is little justification for a segregation of the syndrome from migraine and its variants, he did not fully commit himself. He chose the title of "A particular variety of headache" for his paper. He advocated treatment with daily injections of ergotamine tartrate — a therapy which is often effective when all else has failed — and points out that these injections may be given over long periods without any serious toxic effects. Further reference to these observations will be made in Chapter 7.

This writer has seen some 70 patients with cluster headache over a period of 25 years. The following case history provides a typical example.

A solicitor, aged 27 years, was referred in March, 1979. He had suffered from clusters of severe unilateral headache for eight years. They occurred about twice each year; he had not noted any circumstances in his environment which contributed to them. Each cluster continued for three to four weeks. Before the last bout, which began in December, 1978, he had only one attack each day and this occurred regularly at 10am. In the last bout, two paroxysms distressed him every day: the first at 3am and the second at 7am. A very severe, throbbing pain was always confined to the left supraorbital region and was associated with mild photophobia, but not with any other disturbance of vision or nausea. Each attack of pain lasted for 60 to 90 minutes. During that time there was profuse lacrimation of the left eye as well as a watery discharge from the left nostril which felt "stuffy". In the long intervals between his clusters he felt perfectly well and never had a headache. He had no past history of migraine, allergy or bilious attacks and no family history of migraine was known. Neurological and general physical examination showed no abnormality.

A chronic variant of cluster headache was described during the past ten years, though sporadic cases had been reported in the literature before then. The intensity, situation and duration of pain and the accompanying lacrimation and nasal congestion are identical to cluster headache, but the attacks lose their periodicity and continue to occur daily or haphazardly for several months or years. One of the patients described in some detail by Symonds (1956a) suffered daily attacks over a period of 14 months, but could prevent them by giving himself an injection of ergotamine tartrate each night and morning. The attacks recurred when he ceased these injections. Five patients with "chronic symptoms" were included in a series of 105 patients with cluster headache described by Ekbom (1970). Ekbom subdivided these into two types: a primary chronic type where the patient had no preceding history of shorter cluster headaches and a secondary chronic type where many years of cluster headaches with long remissions were later replaced by the chronic syndrome. Several papers published during the last ten years have pointed out that the chronic forms of cluster headache do not respond as favourably to ergotamines and methysergide as the periodic remitting type, quite apart from the fact that sustained use of large doses of these drugs is undesirable and fraught with risks of toxic effects. As the condition is rare, the number of patients treated is small. However Kudrow (1978) has shown that lithium carbonate is the drug of choice for the treatment of the chronic syndrome. This view is shared by Pearce (1980) who used the title "chronic migrainous neuralgia" if the duration of a cluster was longer than four months. In the absence of bouts separated by remissions, the term chronic cluster headache implies a contradiction of the concept of cluster. The title of chronic migrainous neuralgia is also open to criticism as the migrainous basis of the syndrome is not universally accepted. In Pearce's series of 101 patients with cluster headache, six had the chronic syndrome. In four of these, it developed after a previous history of clusters. It is likely that chronic migrainous neuralgia is more common than currently available reports would indicate and that the condition is frequently misdiagnosed.

The importance of early recognition lies in the potential success of correct treatment. The following case history may help to illustrate this.

A 62-year-old business executive was first seen in June, 1976, with a history of bouts of severe left periorbital and facial pain during the preceding six years. The clusters initially lasted for a few weeks and were separated by intervals of three months of complete freedom from pain. The duration of his remissions diminished gradually; in 1976, it never exceeded two to three weeks. The vast majority of attacks was nocturnal, usually beginning within 90 minutes of falling asleep and recurring two to four times during the night. Each paroxysm lasted for from five to 30 minutes. He described it as a devastating, burning pain confined to the left eyebrow and periorbital area during the first five years of his illness; later, it spread to involve the forehead, cheek, mastoid region and mandible on the left side. The pain was always associated with watering of the left eye and with a clear discharge from the left nostril. The right half of his head or face was never involved. He had been investigated and treated for sinusitis by an otorhinolaryngological surgeon and for three months had taken large doses of carbamazepine on the erroneous diagnosis of trigeminal neuralgia, but he obtained no relief. He had never suffered from headaches before the age of 56 years and had no family history of migraine. Neurological examination did not show Horner's syndrome or any other abnormality. Treatment with methysergide and ergotamine tartrate each night completely prevented his attacks, but the pain recurred if he did not take this medication. The doses were gradually reduced and he enjoyed a remission of 14 months. During the next nine months, he suffered three more clusters, each lasting for from four to six weeks. The attacks were again nocturnal and no longer responded to adequate doses of ergotamine tartrate and methysergide. In May, 1978, a course of treatment with prednisone quickly controlled his attacks. During the last six months of 1978, he had two further bouts and each was rapidly curtailed by prednisone, taken together with methysergide and ergotamine tartrate. After a free interval of eight months, a further cluster persisted for six weeks in spite of the same treatment. The next bout, with symptoms identical to those he had experienced in all previous attacks, began in March, 1980, and continued for the next five months in spite of treatment. He had one or several paroxysms of pain each night, unrelieved by strong analgesics and by a further course of prednisone, but eventually controlled by injections of dihydro-ergotamine which he administered to himself each night.

Cluster headache and its chronic variant were described in greater detail than their apparent rarity may appear to warrant. The clinical features are so characteristic, even stereotyped, that the diagnosis is easy for any physician who is aware of the condition. The differential diagnosis from trigeminal neuralgia, temporal arteritis, infection or neoplasm of the paranasal sinuses, glaucoma and "atypical" facial neuralgias will be described in more detail in Chapter 6. Table I summarizes the essential clinical features which differentiate cluster headache from common and classic migraine. It shows that there are more differences than similarities and that the main common denominator is the therapeutic response to vasoconstrictor drugs. The pain of cluster headache is certainly related to changes in vascular tone. The occurrence of distinct clusters, the occasional clockwork regularity of paroxysms, the periorbital and strictly unilateral situation of pain and the lacrimation and nasal congestion associated with it remain an enigma. Only when the mechanisms underlying these remarkable clinical features are explained will we be able to decide if cluster headache is a migraine variant or not.

Migraine Equivalents

Symptoms indicative of disturbed autonomic regulation in various parts of the body appear to be more prevalent in sufferers of common migraine than in the general population. These include vasomotor dizziness, episodes of palpitations, poor adaptation to climatic changes in the peripheral circulation, pains in the chest attributed to coronary angiospasm, dysmenorrhoea, and episodes of abdominal pain for which no pathological lesion of the abdominal viscera can

Table I. Summary of clinical features which differentiate cluster headache from common and classic migraine.

Features	Cluster headache	Common migraine	Classic migraine
Family history	Very rare; less than 1%	50–75%	Less than 50%
Timing in bouts	Yes	No	No
Number of pain paroxysms	1–6 per 24 hours	Less than 1 per week	Less than 1 per month
Duration of pain	Average of 30–120 minutes	Average of 12–24 hours	Average of less than 12 hours
Site of pain	Unilateral periorbital, spreading to face and temple	Alternating sides of hemicrania or holocrania	Often hemicranial, but side changes in different attacks
Visual or sensory prodromata	Almost never	Uncommon	Common
Nausea and vomiting	Very rare	Very common	Fairly common
Lacrimation and nasal congestion on side of pain	Usual	Almost never	Very rare
Response to ergotamines and methysergide	Often very good	Occasionally good	Frequently good
Plasma serotonin during pain	No change	Falls	Falls
Whole blood histamine during pain	Rises	No change	No change

be demonstrated. For the latter, the term "abdominal migraine" has been used for over a century since Liveing (1873) included such a patient in his monograph on *Megrim, Sick Headache and Some Allied Disorders.*

Abdominal Migraine

While the significance of a past history of "cyclic vomiting" or of the "recurrent syndrome" during the childhood of adult migraineurs is widely recognized (Waters, 1972), there is some scepticism about the validity of a concept of abdominal migraine. Lundberg (1978) provides evidence that recurrent attacks of abdominal pain of specific type may occur in some migraine patients and suggests that a diagnosis of abdominal migraine can be made from the following criteria.

1. A history of classic or common migraine in the patient and/or a family history of migraine.

2. Recurrent, stereotyped attacks of abdominal pain, lasting from one to several hours, and usually located in the upper part of the abdomen.

3. No abdominal symptoms between attacks.

4. Beginning of attacks of abdominal pain in childhood or early adult life.

Recurrent attacks of abdominal pain occur far more often in migrainous children than in adults with migraine. Bille (1962) found that 15 of 73 children (20.5%), aged from 9 to 15 years, with definite migraine also complained of paroxysmal pain in the abdomen. Only one of these continued to have similar attacks of abdominal pain after 16 years of age (cited by Lundberg, 1978). In a series of 100 adult migraineurs, Lundberg (1978) found 12 with abdominal migraine in contrast to only one of 100 patients with muscle contraction headache. However, such a high incidence of abdominal migraine has not been reported by others in the voluminous literature on migraine. It has also not been this writer's experience.

A diagnosis of abdominal migraine in adults should be considered if recurrent attacks of upper abdominal pain occur in patients with more conventional symptoms of migraine and particularly if the abdominal discomfort is preceded by or associated with headache. There is a female preponderance and most patients will provide a history of similar attacks since childhood or early adult life. The abdominal pain usually continues for from one to six hours and is not relieved by taking food, antacids and anticholinergic drugs. It may respond to treatment with orally or parenterally administered ergotamines.

The pathophysiological mechanisms of abdominal migraine have not been fully elucidated. In view of the widespread dysregulation of the autonomic nervous system, gastric atony and stasis, delayed gastric emptying and abnormal motility of the bile ducts, as well as excessive distension of the intra-abdominal arteries and arterioles similar to that which occurs in the extracranial vessels, were considered.

Although the existence of abdominal migraine, particularly in children, can hardly be denied, great care must be exercised in making this diagnosis. There are so many varieties and causes of abdominal pain that migraine should not be considered in either adults or children unless the patient also suffers from more typical symptoms of migraine and until all other pathological processes in the abdomen which may need surgical attention have been excluded by appropriate investigations.

Benign Sex Headache

Severe headaches of short duration which appear acutely during sexual intercourse, particularly at the time of orgasm, have been the subject of a few reports in the literature during the past 25 years. As subarachnoid haemorrhage caused by a ruptured intracranial aneurysm may also occur during sexual activity, it is important to distinguish the benign and brief "sex headache" from the more serious and protracted headaches, usually associated with vomiting and neck rigidity, which result from intracranial bleeding. Lance (1976) has collected a series of 21 cases and proposed the descriptive term of "benign sex headache". It occurs in both men and women and appears to be related more to sexual excitement than physical exertion. The headache is very severe and mostly occipital or nuchal, but it can radiate forward towards the frontal regions and may then be generalized or unilateral. In most patients, it persists for two to ten minutes only, but often a milder headache continues for the next one to 48 hours. It is not accompanied by any visual disturbance and only rarely by nausea. The duration of pain is shorter if intercourse is interrupted before orgasm. Lance (1976) proposes that the first component of this headache is caused by excessive contraction of the suboccipital and scalp muscles during sexual excitement. Some patients can curtail it by deliberate relaxation. The second component of this headache occurs during orgasm and may be caused by a hyperdynamic circulatory state, as a significant rise in both heart rate and blood pressure at the moment of orgasm was demonstrated in several studies. Examination of the cerebrospinal fluid and cerebral angiography showed no abnormality. The pain does not occur during every intercourse and usually abates spontaneously, but it may recur after months or years.

It is questionable whether "benign sex headache" should be regarded as a migraine equivalent. The second component defined by Lance (1976) appears to be vascular and could include relaxation of extracranial vessels, but the condition has more similarity to the headache which occurs in paroxysmal hypertension due to phaeochromocytoma than to migraine. Only about 25% of the patients reported in the literature, or seen by the writer of this book, have either a personal or family history of migraine.

The occurrence of severe headache during sexual activity creates great emotional distress and may lead to considerable anxiety during subsequent coitus. This can be relieved only by patient explanation from a physician acquainted with the condition. It is for this reason that "benign sex headache" is included in this chapter, even though its place as a migraine equivalent is dubious. The following case history will help to acquaint the reader with a condition which may be more common than reports in the literature suggest.

A 54-year-old business executive had three attacks of short, but very intense, transnuchal headache over a period of six days. Each occurred during coitus and just before orgasm; the intense pain continued for one to two minutes only, but a milder transfrontal headache persisted during the next 12 hours. His vision was not disturbed and he did not feel bilious. During the following week this headache did not recur, although he was apprehensive about it during intercourse. In the past he had suffered only from infrequent frontal headaches at times of stress. His general health was excellent and no family history of migraine was known. Neurological examination was unremarkable and blood pressure was normal.

While in this patient the diagnostic concept of migraine equivalent would hardly be applicable, I have records of other patients with similar sudden and severe headache during sexual activity who had suffered from migraine at other times. One man even had an isolated attack of complicated migraine during intercourse, when an excruciatingly severe occipital headache was accompanied by loss of vision in the right eye and by weakness and paraesthesia of the right limbs. He recovered completely within 40 minutes and thorough investigation, including examination of the cerebrospinal fluid and cerebral angiography, showed no abnormality. We can conclude that the events during some attacks of "benign sex headache" indicate a vascular component, while, in the majority of instances, excessive muscle contraction is the essential pathogenetic mechanism.

Dr Whisnant and his colleagues at the Mayo Clinic (personal communication) observed that "benign sex headache" can often be prevented by a single prophylactic dose of indomethacin or of a compound preparation of ergotamine tartrate and caffeine.

Cough Headache

Although a severe bout of coughing raises intracranial pressure and may cause displacement of intracranial contents towards the foramen magnum and traction on pain-sensitive dural and vascular structures, it is not usually associated with headache. In patients with intracranial space-occupying lesions (particularly in the posterior cranial fossa) and in those with Paget's disease and basilar impression, coughing as well as sneezing, laughing, stooping and lifting weights may produce headache of great severity and short duration. The pain is generalized, frontal, vertical and occipital and usually lasts for a few minutes only. It occurs in patients with normal intracranial pressure in spite of a known or later proven space-occupying lesion and it is attributed to a temporarily diminished venous return and consequent intracranial venous distension with a shift and traction on pain sensitive intracranial structures.

Symonds (1956b) reported a series of 21 patients with transient, very severe, generalized vertical or bifrontal headache, triggered by coughing, sneezing, stooping and straining. The headache lasted from two to ten minutes and was not accompanied by nausea, visual disturbances or focal cerebral symptoms. None had signs of an intracranial expanding lesion during follow-up over many years and nine of them recovered spontaneously. Some had other non-specific spontaneous headaches, unrelated to coughing, but others had not complained of cephalgia before the onset of cough headache. In four patients, the cough headache occurred only in an upright posture. The mechanism of this pure cough headache is unknown, though sudden intracranial or extracranial vascular distension may have a pathogenetic role. Only five (24%) of Symonds' (1956b) cases had a past history of migraine, which casts doubt on the inclusion of this entity as a migraine equivalent. It is mentioned and illustrated by the following case history to draw attention to the fact that not all headaches produced by coughing are due to sinister intracranial lesions.

A businessman, aged 50 years, presented with a history of frequently recurring, but very brief, headaches for two months. He had never suffered from headache before. The headaches were always brought on by coughing, sneezing, stooping or straining. They came on suddenly, and lasted for up to one minute only. The pain was intense and was felt over the vertex and in both temples. It was never associated with any visual symptoms or nausea. He was able to reduce the severity of pain by pressing his palms firmly on his temples whenever he coughed or stooped. No family history of migraine was known. Neurological examination revealed no abnormality and blood pressure was 18.7/12kPa (140/90mm Hg). Treatment with a compound preparation containing 0.3mg of ergotamine tartrate prevented or reduced the severity of his headaches. They disappeared after a further two months. When he was seen again 20 years later the cough headaches had not returned and he was generally well.

This man's observation that his headache could be improved by compressing his superficial temporal arteries, and his favourable response to treatment with a small dose of ergotamine suggest that distension of extracranial arteries contributed to his momentary paroxysms of severe pain in the head whenever he coughed, sneezed or strained.

Migraine in Children

Although the prevalence of migraine during childhood is lower than in adult life, it is by no means uncommon. It increases from 1% below the age of six years to 4.5% of children 10 to 12 years old and to 5.3% at the age of 15 years (Vahlquist, 1955; Bille, 1962). In a series of 8993 Swedish schoolchildren, aged from seven to 15 years, 3.9% suffered from genuine migraine (Bille, 1968). The criteria used for a diagnosis of migraine included a history of paroxysmal headaches separated by free intervals and at least two of the following clinical features: unilateral pain; nausea; visual aura; family history (parents or siblings).

In various large series of adult migraineurs reported in the literature, an onset before the age of 10 years has been reported in from 12% to 30% of cases (Balyeat and Rinkel, 1931; Krayenbühl and Heyck, 1955; Selby and Lance, 1960). Diagnosis in infancy is difficult because the small child cannot communicate his complaints clearly, but many children are able to indicate the location of their distress in the head before they are three years old. A male preponderance in early childhood changes after the age of seven to 10 years, when girls outnumber boys in a ratio of 6 : 4.

Heredity is the most important aetiological factor and Bille (1968) found that children inherit migraine much more often from their mothers (72.6%) than fathers (20.5%). Many children with migraine are said to be intelligent, polite, meticulous and striving to please, but these personality traits were never subjected to statistical analysis.

Some children show other manifestations of autonomic instability such as travel sickness, cyclic vomiting or dizziness. The precipitating factors are similar to those observed in many adults with common migraine and include stress at school, examinations, and even the pleasant excitement and anticipation of a party. Many children have their attacks after playing games at school, particularly on hot and sunny days, and some develop their headaches almost invariably after attending a movie matinee. The frequency of attacks tends to decline during the school vacation.

In children, attacks of migraine occur more often, but are much shorter than in adults. They usually continue for a few hours only and rarely last for 12 hours or longer. Common migraine far exceeds classic migraine during childhood. Apart from irritability and yawning, an aura is unusual. If premonitory symptoms occur, they tend to be visual rather than sensory. Between the ages of seven and nine years only 51% of migrainous children complained of unilateral headache, but the incidence of hemicrania increased to 72% in the age group from 13 to 15 years (Bille, 1968). The most common site of headache is frontal and retro-orbital. The pain is accompanied by nausea in about four out of five migraine attacks and vomiting is only a little less common. Photophobia is next in frequency of associated symptoms, while dizziness, syncope and transient motor and sensory symptoms are relatively rare. A past or concurrent history of epileptic seizures is said to be more common in children with migraine than in those without it, but this view has not yet been supported by statistical studies on large series of patients.

In this author's experience, a common sequence of events is a mild frontal headache which begins on the way home from school in the afternoon, often after rushing about playing sport on a bright and sunny day. The headache increases progressively in severity. Instead of having a glass of milk and a biscuit and then settling down to homework, the child prefers to go to bed in a darkened room. They then sleep for two to three hours, by which time they may have recovered sufficiently to eat their dinner; or else they continue to sleep through the night, but feel perfectly well and fit for school on the following morning. Simple analgesics, such as aspirin, provide some relief unless the child feels bilious and vomits early in the attack.

Cluster headaches and all varieties of complicated migraine, with the exception of rare instances of familial hemiplegic migraine, occur rarely in childhood.

There is a relatively higher incidence of abnormal electroencephalographic tracings in migrainous children than in adults. This may be due partly to the frequent occurrence of non-specific slow activity in children with migraine as well as in those without it, and to the relative difficulty in defining the limits of "normality" in the electroencephalographic tracings recorded from children. We shall refer to this in more detail in the next chapter.

Although results of large prospective studies that have been continued over many years are not available, about one-third of children with migraine tend to become free of attacks before reaching puberty, and a further one-third complain of migraine rarely and infrequently during early adult life. When reviewed after an interval of from nine to 14 years from the diagnosis of migraine in childhood, almost 80% of 58 patients were well or much improved; only 20% were unimproved or worse. Therefore, it would appear that the prognosis of migraine in childhood is better than one would anticipate (Hinrichs and Keith, 1965).

Chapter 5

Assessment and Investigation of the Patient with Migraine

History Taking and Neurological Examination

The diagnosis of migraine rests on taking a meticulous history, because headaches, as well as most associated symptoms, are subjective. Abnormal neurological signs will rarely be found; if they are, it is usually during an attack. The discovery of objective neurological abnormalities in the interval between attacks should cast doubt on a diagnosis of any variant of migraine and establish a need for further investigation.

Family physicians may be summoned to the patient's home at the time of the first attack or if headache and vomiting are severe. However, physicians will be more often consulted at the surgery by patients who seek relief from recurrent headaches interfering with their activities and enjoyment of life. If the patient is seen at home, distraught by pain, photophobia and gastrointestinal complaints, the opportunity for history taking is limited and hence the emphasis should be on excluding acute intracranial lesions which may demand urgent admission to hospital.

The first consideration is the possibility of meningitis, encephalitis, or subarachnoid haemorrhage. Fever, photophobia, pain on eye movement, neck rigidity and a positive Kernig's sign point to an intracranial infection requiring the patient's admission to hospital and examination of the cerebrospinal fluid. The sudden onset of extremely severe sub-occipital or generalized headache, usually associated with vomiting and occasionally with an impaired level of awareness, should arouse suspicion of subarachnoid bleeding. There may be no neck rigidity during the first 24 hours after a subarachnoid haemorrhage; abnormal neurological signs are often conspicuous by their absence. It is essential to examine the optic fundi with an ophthalmoscope as subhyaloid haemorrhages, though uncommon, will immediately establish the correct diagnosis. The patient should be admitted to hospital as soon as possible so that the cerebrospinal fluid can be examined and the diagnosis confirmed or excluded. A history of a recent, perhaps trivial, head injury must arouse thoughts of an extradural or subdural haematoma, even in the absence of papilloedema and of abnormal focal neurological signs. This is a treacherous condition which should always be in the physician's mind, particularly if the headache is progressing in severity and is associated with a declining level of consciousness and an inequality of the size of the pupils. A high level of suspicion and admission to a hospital with facilities for appropriate investigations may save the patient's life. With the exception of some tumours in the posterior cranial fossa and the less common intraventricular lesions (such as colloid cysts of the third ventricle which obstruct the outflow of cerebrospinal fluid) it is unusual for cerebral tumours to cause acute headache of sufficient severity to demand a home consultation.

After these acute medical emergencies have been excluded, the possibility of tension (muscle contraction) headache or of migraine should be assessed by specific inquiry for the following.

A. A previous history of similar or other headaches.
B. Family history of migraine.
C. Symptoms, if any, of an aura preceding the headache.
D. Situation of pain — hemicranial or generalized.
E. Associated visual symptoms — blurring, teichopsia or photophobia.
F. Focal sensory, motor or speech disturbances.
G. Dizziness and faintness.
H. Gastrointestinal complaints, including anorexia, nausea, vomiting and diarrhoea.
I. Tenderness of the scalp.
J. Environmental events which may have precipitated the attack.
K. The patient's personality — tense, depressed or obsessional.

A full neurological examination and a general physical examination are mandatory. Abnormal neurological findings, such as ptosis, expressive dysphasia, slight weakness of limbs or minor sensory impairment, may be found in classic or complicated migraine, but the patient should be examined again on the following day to determine if these signs have resolved. Slight fever and even mild neck stiffness occur occasionally during an episode of severe migraine. The distinction from a viral meningoencephalitis can then be made only by examining the patient again after a few hours, before deciding on the necessity for lumbar puncture and examination of the cerebrospinal fluid.

The information gained from the history and examination, the observations of the patient's behaviour and a previous knowledge or assessment of personality traits usually provide adequate information for a distinction between migraine and tension (muscle contraction) headache. It is advisable to invite the patient to come to the surgery after recovery from the acute attack. Here, a decision can be made on the need for laboratory investigations and therapeutic measures can be recommended to reduce the risk of recurrence.

A more leisurely approach can be adopted when the patient seeks treatment for chronic or recurrent headaches in the family physician's surgery. The doctor's task is now to distinguish migraine from other chronic and potentially serious causes of headache such as: infections of the paranasal sinuses; ocular disorders; excessive muscle contraction due to anxiety; hypertension and cerebral vascular disease; temporal arteritis; and subacute or chronic intracranial space-occupying lesions.

A detailed history always provides the best diagnostic information; an average of 15 minutes should be allocated to this. The essential criterion for a diagnosis of migraine is the *paroxysmal occurrence* of headache. If at least two of the following clinical features are also present, the diagnosis can be made with more confidence.

A. A family history of migraine in parents or siblings.
B. Precipitation of some attacks by environmental factors, including stress, glare, certain foods and menstruation.
C. A visual or sensory aura preceding the headache.
D. Unilateral situation of pain.
E. Anorexia, nausea, vomiting and other gastrointestinal complaints.
F. Tenderness of the scalp.

However, a more detailed history will not only increase diagnostic accuracy, but may also discover aetiological factors applicable to individual patients and may contribute to more successful treatment of their migraine. An adequate history should aim to elicit the following information.

Information to obtain from patients.
A. Date of the first episode of similar headache.
B. Average frequency of attacks per week, month or year.
C. Usual time of onset of headache.
D. Range of duration of attacks.
E. Severity and character of pain — dull, throbbing or "splitting".
F. Situation of pain — hemicranial or generalized.
G. If hemicranial, does it always involve the same side?
H. Premonitory symptoms and their duration — visual, sensory or other.
I. Photophobia during the attack.
J. Intolerance to noise or to odours.
K. Associated gastrointestinal complaints, including anorexia, nausea, vomiting and diarrhoea. How long after the onset of headache do these occur?
L. Disorders of movement, sensation or speech before or during the headache. Are the motor or sensory disorders on the same side or opposite to the side of hemicrania?
M. Dizziness, faintness or transient loss of consciousness.
N. Are the headache and accompanying complaints of sufficient severity to demand cessation of work and activities, or confinement to bed?
O. A feeling of lassitude or exhaustion at the end of the attack.
P. What treatment was previously tried either for prevention or for the acute attack? How effective was it?
Q. Relationship of the attacks to environmental stress, climate, glare, or to specific foods or beverages.
R. In female patients, do the attacks occur only in relation to the menstrual cycle or are they more frequent and severe before, during or after menstruation?
S. Is the patient taking oral contraceptives and have these had any influence on the frequency and severity of her migraine?
T. The patient's personality traits — unable to relax, prone to worry, tense, tidy, meticulous or obsessional.
U. A past history of similar headaches earlier in life.
V. A history of bilious attacks or travel sickness in childhood.
W. A past or concurrent history of allergic disorders, including hay fever, urticaria and asthma.
X. A family history of migraine in parents, siblings or the patient's children.

It is also important to ascertain whether the headaches have recently changed in frequency, situation or severity so that the possibility of a more serious intracranial lesion in a previously migrainous patient is not overlooked.

Family physicians who care for a large population of headache patients may find it more convenient to use a questionnaire which may be completed at the time of the consultation or handed to the patient before or after the consultation. An example of such a questionnaire is provided, which can be modified or abbreviated according to the individual physician's need.

Headache Questionnaire

Name ....

Date of birth ....

Date of consultation ....

Please answer all questions. With the exception of questions 3, 9, 18 and 20 a simple tick or cross for the alternative which applies to you suffices as an answer.

1. Do your headaches occur
   A. every day for weeks or months?   ....
   B. in recurrent attacks lasting hours or days?   ....

2. How long have you suffered from headaches?
   A. a few weeks or months.   ....
   B. more than one year.   ....
   C. more than five years.   ....

3. On an average, how many attacks of headache do you have
   A. per week?   ....
   B. per month?   ....
   C. per year?   ....

4. Do your headaches usually begin
   A. during the night?   ....
   B. on waking?   ....
   C. any time of day?   ....

5. What is the average duration of headache?
   A. a few hours.   ....
   B. all day.   ....
   C. several days.   ....

6. Describe the character of your pain
   A. dull.   ....
   B. throbbing.   ....
   C. splitting.   ....

7. Where is the pain situated?
   A. all over the head.   ....
   B. across the forehead.   ....
   C. mainly at the back of the head.   ....
   D. always on one side of the head.   ....
   E. worse on one side of the head.   ....

8. If the pain is always on one side, is it consistently
    A. on the same side? ....
    B. right side? ....
    C. left side? ....

9. If you have a warning before your headache, does it consist of
    A. blurring of vision? ....
    B. shimmering lights, circles, other shapes or colours? ....
    C. numbness of lips, tongue, fingers or legs? ....
    D. other warning symptoms? ....

10. How long do these warning symptoms last?
    A. less than 20 minutes. ....
    B. 20 minutes to an hour. ....
    C. an hour or longer. ....

11. Is the headache accompanied by
    A. intolerance of light? ....
    B. intolerance of noise? ....
    C. sensitivity to odours? ....

12. During the attack of headache do you
    A. lose your appetite? ....
    B. feel bilious? ....
    C. vomit? ....
    D. have diarrhoea? ....

13. If you vomit, does this usually occur
    A. within an hour from the onset of headache? ....
    B. after two hours? ....
    C. after several hours? ....

14. During the attack of headache do you experience
    A. numbness or pins and needles of lips, tongue, fingers, legs? ....
    B. weakness of limbs? ....
    C. numbness or weakness on the same side as the headache? ....
    D. numbness on the opposite side to the headache? ....
    E. difficulty in finding words or other disturbances of your speech? ....
    F. dizziness? ....
    G. blackouts? ....

15. Are the headaches usually so severe that
    A. you cannot perform your work or other activities? ....
    B. you must go to bed? ....

16. At the end of an attack of headache do you feel
    A. tired, listless or exhausted? ....
    B. relieved and exhilarated? ....

17. What treatment have you had for your headaches in the past?
    A. aspirin and similar pain-relieving drugs. ....
    B. ergot preparations (such as Cafergot, Ergodryl or Migral). ....
    C. medications to relieve biliousness. ....
    D. injections of strong pain-relieving drugs. ....
    E. sedatives or tranquillizing drugs. ....

18. Have you taken any medication for the prevention of your attacks?
If so, do you know the name of the medication?

....

19. Was the medication for prevention or for treatment of the acute attack
successful   ....
A. completely?   ....
B. partly?   ....
C. not at all?

20. Have you recognized any circumstances in your environment which will
bring on an attack, such as
A. emotional stress or excitement?   ....
B. climate (for example, heat and humidity)?   ....
C. exposure to glare or flickering light?   ....
D. foods or beverages (for example, chocolate, fried foods, oranges, spir-
its, red or white wine — please state which of these applies to you) ?
                                                                                                         ....

The next two questions apply to female patients only:

21. Do your attacks occur
A. only in association with menstruation?   ....
B. if so, are they worse before, during or just after your periods   ....

22. If you are taking a contraceptive pill, did this affect the frequency and
severity of your headaches?   ....
A. did they improve?   ....
B. did they become worse?

23. How would you assess your personality?
A. calm.   ....
B. unable to relax.   ....
C. tense and a worrier.   ....
D. meticulous and very tidy.   ....

24. During childhood did you suffer from
A. occasional headaches?   ....
B. bilious attacks?   ....
C. travel sickness?   ....
D. convulsions?   ....

25. Did you suffer from allergic complaints such as
A. hay fever?   ....
B. hives?   ....
C. asthma?   ....

26. Does anyone in your family suffer from headaches similar to yours?
A. parents.   ....
B. brothers or sisters.   ....
C. children.   ....

It is not always easy to obtain clear and decisive answers to all these questions from anxious and talkative patients, but many will co-operate if it is pointed out that correct answers will help materially in the better treatment of their complaint. In addition to diagnostic and aetiological information, the questions are designed to assist in a therapeutic strategy. The frequency of attacks will determine the need for sustained prophylactic treatment; the usual time of onset helps to select the timing of doses; the occurrence of vomiting within an hour after the onset of headache will imply that any oral drug treatment for the acute attack is destined to fail. Many of the common precipitating factors can be avoided. Intelligent patients should be encouraged to write down events which may have contributed to each attack before their next visit to the doctor.

If the answer to the initial questions concerning frequency, periodicity and duration of headache suggests the possibility of cluster headache, this should be pursued by seeking answers to further specific questions such as:

A. History of previous bouts (clusters) and their duration.
B. Number of attacks during 24 hours.
C. Timing of attacks.
D. Duration of attacks.
E. Situation of pain and any change from side to side during a single cluster.
F. Lacrimation of the eye on the side of headache.
G. Clear discharge from a stuffy nostril on the same side.
H. Occurrence of ptosis on the side of pain.
I. Presence or absence of visual disturbances.

Some of the more dramatic symptoms of migraine variants, though relatively uncommon, are prone to arouse suspicion of a more serious vascular or expanding intracranial lesion. Physicians' knowledge of the characteristic clinical features (described in Chapter 4) should help them to formulate specific questions designed to test the possibility of a migrainous aetiology. A diagnosis of complicated migraine should be considered if there is a past history of: similar transient disorders of vision or pareses of ocular muscles; episodes of hemiparesis; headache, with or without nausea, associated with some of the visual or cerebral symptoms; attacks of common or classic migraine; and if there is a family history of migraine of a similar or different type.

Migraine without headache often presents diagnostic difficulties. A positive family history, or a past personal history of common or classic migraine is helpful, though not essential. A careful description of the episodic occurrence, duration and nature of the visual disturbance, or of the clinical features associated with attacks of vertigo, should allow the physician to consider this diagnosis and to determine the need for further investigations.

Even though a detailed history usually provides essential diagnostic clues, adequate neurological and general examinations must be performed. This will give the physician confidence that a more serious intracranial lesion has not been overlooked. It will help also to assure the patient that no effort was spared to make a diagnosis and to provide appropriate treatment. With a little practice and a planned programme, a full neurological examination can be performed in less than 10 minutes.

The following programme is recommended:

Programme for neurological examination

1. Ophthalmoscopic examination of optic discs, retinae and retinal vessels.
2. Visual fields by confrontation.
3. Pupils and their reactions.
4. External ocular movements.
5. Survey of other cranial nerves.
6. Muscle tone, power and co-ordination of all limbs.
7. Brief sensory examination, mainly of cortical sensation (passive movement of fingers, stereognosis). More detailed sensory testing is necessary only if migraine attacks include sensory symptoms.
8. Tendon reflexes in upper and lower limbs. The plantar responses need to be elicited only if there is a history of hemiparesis or if the tendon reflexes are asymmetrical.
9. Stance and gait.
10. Listen for a bruit over the orbits. The bell of the stethoscope is applied over one eye, while both eyes are shut. If the patient is then asked to open the other eye and look up, the confusing noise of fluttering eyelids can be eliminated or at least reduced. It is easier to hear a soft bruit if examiners also keep their fingers on the radial pulse, as an intracranial bruit is synchronous with the pulse beat. In children under the age of 10 years, a bruit heard either over one or both orbits usually has no pathological significance.
11. Palpation of the superficial temporal arteries. These arteries sometimes remain tender on the side of hemicrania for some days after an attack of migraine. A swollen, hard and very tender temporal artery should suggest the possibility of temporal arteritis.
12. Record blood pressure.

The heart, chest and abdomen should also be examined. Such examination should always be performed on the first visit of a patient who complains of headache and who is not well known to the family physician.

Visual, sensory or motor symptoms during an attack of classic or complicated migraine will require more thorough examination of the eyes or limbs.

In the majority of patients, a detailed history and physical examination will allow the physician to make a confident and correct diagnosis of migraine. Laboratory investigations are needed only if some doubt remains about the possibility of structural cerebral pathology, such as an arteriovenous malformation or other vascular or expanding lesion. These investigations are also needed if the nature of the patient's blackouts is uncertain, or if a very apprehensive patient requires the graphic proof that the headaches and associated symptoms are not due to a tumour or some other serious intracranial mischief.

Plain X-ray Examinations

Skull X-ray examinations have no value in the investigation of migraine and its variants. The very rare instances of calcification in a vascular malformation or tumour, or displacement of a calcified pineal gland, would be demonstrated more convincingly by abnormal uptake of isotope in a nuclear brain scan, or by the even more informative changes in a computerized tomographic brain scan. However, these tests should be performed only if there are good clinical indications or if the patient demands them for peace of mind. Pituitary tumours do not cause episodic headaches similar to migraine; X-ray examinations of the pituitary fossa should be ordered only if symptoms of endocrine dysfunction and defects of the visual fields point to the possibility of a pituitary neoplasm.

X-ray examinations of the paranasal sinuses are required only if the patient has suffered from recurrent sinus infections, has a chronic nasal discharge, and is tender to pressure on the frontal or maxillary sinuses. It is amazing how often patients with obvious common migraine present to the neurologist after years of unsuccessful treatment for chronic sinusitis.

Radiological examination of the cervical spine is not only of no use in the investigation of migraine, but can be misleading. Degenerative changes in the cervical vertebrae and their joints, osteophytes and the narrowing of cervical disc spaces are as common and as physiological in patients over the age of 50 years as grey hair. Even if the migrainous headaches begin in the suboccipital or occipital region and the patient's range of neck movement is reduced, this degenerative cervical spondylosis cannot cause episodic migrainous headaches with the usual visual and gastrointestinal accompaniments. The short-sighted, but vocal, enthusiasm of neck manipulators, who claim to cure almost all patients with migraine, has not been confirmed by the experience of most physicians and neurologists. Chiropractic and other manipulative manoeuvres of the cervical spine can provide temporary respite from muscle contraction (tension) headache, but they have no more than a placebo effect in the treatment of migraine. Therefore, there is no need for radiological examination of the cervical spine in the investigation or treatment of a patient with a history of migraine or allied vascular headache.

Nuclear Brain Scans

The dearth of literature on isotope brain scanning in migraine suggests that this investigation has only a limited indication. In a country town with facilities for nuclear scanning, but geographically remote from computerized tomographic scanners, a static nuclear scan would save expense in providing reassurance for the over-anxious patient. Static isotope scans are reliable in demonstrating arteriovenous malformations or tumours in instances of symptomatic migraine suggested by a history of hemicrania consistently on the same side, associated with contralateral neurological symptoms or with partial (focal) or generalized seizures. Dynamic scans (isotope flow studies) may be of value in the study of patients with classic or complicated migraine, when the headaches are associated with focal retinal or cerebral symptoms. Technological advances are improving the accuracy and increasing the application of such dynamic flow studies and they should soon become a useful research tool for the investigation of both intracranial and extracranial blood flow before and during an attack of migraine. Dynamic nuclear flow studies may also help to elucidate or exclude arterial stenoses in the differentiation of specific cases of complicated migraine from occlusive cerebral vascular disease.

Computerized Tomographic (CT) Brain Scans

The introduction of computerized tomographic (CT) brain scanning is the biggest advance in the diagnostic investigation of cerebral disorders which has occurred this century. It is more informative and more accurate than any other investigation. It is non-invasive and has no adverse effects, but it involves either patients or insurance funds in considerable expense. The taking of an adequate history and neurological examination can achieve a correct diagnosis of migraine in over 95% of cases. Computerized tomographic brain scanning should be reserved for the following.

A. Research of the acute events and chronic residual effects in classic and complicated migraine.

B. Diagnosis of a structural cerebral lesion (vascular or neoplastic) suggested from the history or from abnormal physical signs.

C. Reassurance of the over-anxious patient who has heard about CT scanning from friends or through the media and demands this investigation irrespective of expense.

A number of papers published since 1976 report on the findings of CT brain scans obtained either between or during attacks, or performed to investigate residual visual or neurological deficits attributed to past migrainous episodes. Cala and Mastaglia (1976) describe 46 patients, aged from 17 to 35 years, with a history of severe migraine extending for up to 18 years. They were referred for CT brain scans because of an increasing frequency and severity of migraine attacks. In 12 of them the scan was performed during a headache and 14 patients had persistently abnormal focal neurological signs. The results of only nine scans (19.6%) were completely normal. Twenty-one (45.7%) showed signs of mild cerebral oedema, mainly bifrontal, but the scans of seven of these 21 patients were performed during an attack. The CT scan demonstrated signs of cerebral infarction in six patients (13%): in four of these, the scan confirmed an appropriate persistent defect of the visual field; in the remaining two there were no associated clinical signs. This may be interpreted as evidence of past migrainous ischaemic cerebral infarction. The scans of eight patients (17.4%) had signs of cerebral atrophy, including widening of sulci and fissures and enlarged lateral or third ventricles. The degree of cerebral atrophy was significant in only two patients who had suffered from frequent and severe classic migraine. Tumours were discovered in two patients, but in one of these the history had pointed to such a tumour and demanded further investigation. In a later paper (Cala and Mastaglia, 1980), the same authors had extended the series of migrainous patients to 94, but the incidence of cerebral atrophy dropped to 11.8% and the frequency of oedema declined to 6.4% suggesting that the authors had become more critical in interpreting the CT signs of oedema and atrophy.

A similar study of 53 patients with exceptionally severe migraine, often associated with focal symptoms, was reported by Hungerford, du Boulay and Zilkha (1976). The average age of their patients was 42.7 years and the average duration of migraine since onset was 20 years. All but one of the CT scans were performed between attacks. The results of 28 scans (52.8%) were normal. Only one patient showed curious bilateral areas of decreased density in the cerebral hemispheres, which may have represented oedema. The scans of six patients (11.3%) showed signs of cerebral infarction, either unilateral or bilateral. However, in three of these patients the authors were not certain if migraine was necessarily the sole cause of the infarction. Unequivocal evidence of cerebral atrophy (enlarged ventricles and/or cortical subarachnoid spaces) was found in 14 patients (26.4%): in eight of these the atrophic changes were focal; in six, they were generalized. The incidence of cerebral atrophy in this series is higher than in the patients reported by Cala and Mastaglia (1976,1980). This may be due to the fact that the patients studied by Hungerford *et al.* (1976) were older and may have included a larger proportion of cases with exceptionally severe, chronic and/or hemiplegic migraine. The authors argue that generalized cerebral atrophy (usually mild to moderate) in their patients was probably age related, while the eight instances of focal cerebral atrophy may have resulted from old, mature infarcts. The situation of focal cerebral infarcts was at times in agreement with the patient's history of focal neurological signs during a migrainous aura. There was no association between abnormalities in the results of CT brain scans and treatment with ergot derivatives.

Several reports refer to isolated cases of complicated migraine where CT scan examinations showed cerebral infarction in the appropriate area of the brain. Four cases of cerebral infarction, documented by CT scanning and arteriography, in young migrainous patients aged from 16 to 32 years were reported by Dorfman, Marshall and Enzmann (1979). One of these caused no symptoms relative to the scan lesion, one was associated with mild and transient complaints, and two produced lasting neurological deficits. Other risk factors for ischaemic cerebral vascular disease were fully excluded in two cases. The findings on the CT scans were low density lesions with or without contrast enhancement, no surrounding oedema, and partial or complete resolution of the lesion on later CT examination.

The observations of CT scanning of the brain so far available have confirmed and extended the long held clinical suspicion that focal cerebral infarction may occur, though very infrequently, in classic or complicated migraine. This is most often seen in the territory of the posterior cerebral artery in patients with persistent visual field defects. It remains uncertain whether this infarction is due to focal spasm of small cerebral vessels, to shunting of blood to other parts of the brain, or to changes in platelet aggregation. After many years of recurrent episodes of severe classic migraine, small focal areas of cerebral atrophy may remain as evidence of past infarction although there may be no permanent residual neurological signs.

It must be stressed that the results of CT brain scans cited above were concerned with selected groups of patients and are not representative of the large migraine population in general. Normal CT scans are obtained between attacks from the majority of patients, even from some of those with exceptionally severe classic or complicated migraine. If the investigation can be performed during

Fig. 6. EEG showing slow activity predominating from the left post-central region.

Fig. 7. CT brain scan which shows areas of low density and patchy contrast enhancement in the left frontotemporal region. The body of the left lateral ventricle is severely compressed.

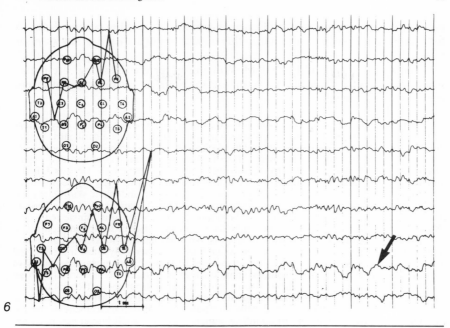

6

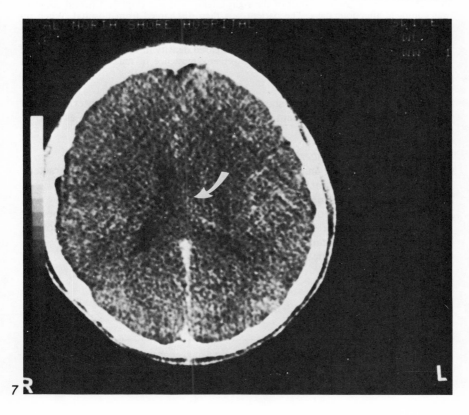

7

the course of an episode of complicated migraine, we would expect evidence of focal cerebral ischaemia or oedema; this should resolve within a few days or weeks.

The author is grateful to Dr P.M. Williamson for the following case report which illustrates the value of CT scanning of the brain for the diagnosis of severe complicated migraine.

A 17-year-old boy who had never suffered from migraine and had no family history of it noted difficulty in moving his right arm and left leg while riding a surfboard. Within minutes he developed a severe generalized headache and nausea and became drowsy. After he arrived home he vomited repeatedly; then he became mentally confused and vague. Weakness of his right arm and left leg recovered within a few hours. He was initially admitted to a hospital in a country town and remained drowsy and slightly confused for three days. The results of full blood count, serum chemistry and plain skull X-ray examinations were normal, but electroencephalography showed marked focal slow activity from the posterior half of the left cerebral hemisphere. The patient was transferred to the Royal North Shore Hospital of Sydney three days after the onset of these symptoms, still complaining of headache, nausea and drowsiness. No abnormalities were found on neurological or general examination. The cerebrospinal fluid contained only a few traumatic red cells, no white cells, a slightly raised protein level of 0.60g/L and normal amounts of glucose and chloride. Electroencephalographic tracings were markedly abnormal with an excess of bilateral, post-central slow activity predominating from the left cerebral hemisphere (Fig. 6). The computerized tomographic brain scan, with and without contrast infusion, showed mixed areas of low density and patchy contrast enhancement in the left frontotemporal region with almost complete compression of the left lateral ventricle, but did not show any significant shift of the right lateral ventricle (Fig. 7). Clinical recovery was complete after four days. The patient was then discharged from hospital. When reviewed four weeks later, he reported that he had remained completely well. The results of a progress electroencephalogram were entirely normal (Fig. 8) and the computerized tomographic brain scan showed only an area of decreased density in the region of the head of the left caudate nucleus. There was no longer any evidence of mass effect or contrast enhancement (Fig. 9).

When should a family or a specialist physician request a computerized tomographic brain scan for a patient with migraine? The indications are as follow.

Indications for computerized tomographic (CT) brain scan
1. A recent, significant change in the frequency, severity or clinical characteristics of migraine attacks.
2. Persistence of focal neurological deficits.
3. Hemicrania always on the same side, associated with contralateral neurological symptoms or signs, or presence of an orbital bruit suggestive of an underlying arteriovenous malformation.
4. History of partial (focal) seizures.

Fig. 8. Progress EEG after four weeks showing return to normal cerebral rhythms.

Fig. 9. Progress CT brain scan after four weeks. The mass effect and areas of contrast enhancement have disappeared and the body of the left lateral ventricle is now normal.

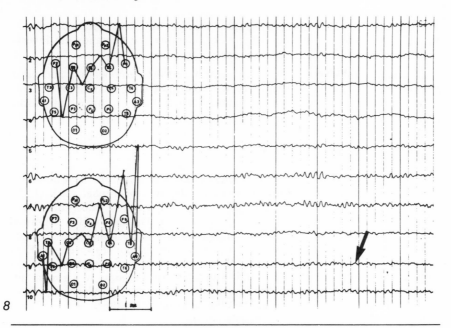

8

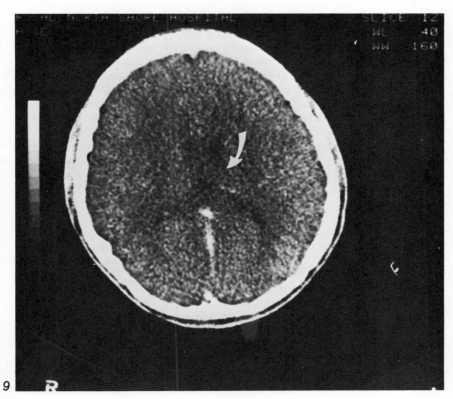

9

5. Unequivocal electroencephalographic evidence of a focal cerebral lesion.
6. A patient who doubts the diagnosis of migraine and demands full investigation before accepting the therapeutic limitations.

Technological advances, such as positron emission tomography and other methods currently under development, will contribute more to an understanding of the vascular events during a migraine attack than to clinical diagnostic accuracy.

Electroencephalography

While the computerized tomographic brain scan provides us with information about structural lesions of the brain, the electroencephalogram (EEG) records abnormalities in the electrical activity of cortical or subcortical areas which cannot always be correlated with clinical events. Some of the abnormal EEG patterns are transient, and it may reasonably be assumed that they are caused by a focal or diffuse reduction in cerebral perfusion. However, the EEG cannot provide positive evidence for this assumption. Unfortunately, it is not often possible to record the EEG during an attack of migraine. In a similar situation to that which applies to the investigation of epilepsy, the highest yield of abnormal EEGs in migraine would be obtained during an attack, yet even then a proportion of tracings will be entirely normal.

A review of the large literature on EEGs recorded in the interval between migraine attacks shows that diffuse or focal abnormalities of various types are more common than in non-migrainous patients. It may be predicted on clinical grounds that EEG abnormalities should be more frequent and more florid in patients with classic and complicated migraine than in those with common migraine. There is no specific EEG pattern diagnostic of migraine. Persistent or episodic slow frequencies, bursts or paroxysms of sharp waves, spikes and even spike and wave complexes (which are more often regarded as indicative of epilepsy) have been found; so have focal slow and sharp waves which are at times, but not always, consistent with focal visual, motor or sensory disorders.

On the basis of paroxysmal activity in the EEG tracings of a small series of patients, Weil (1952) proposed the concept of "dysrhythmic" migraine. Later reports claimed that patients with episodic EEG discharges showed a good response to treatment with hydantoins and other anticonvulsant drugs. These claims were not substantiated and the concept of "dysrhythmic" migraine has been largely abandoned.

Before we can assess the frequency of abnormal EEG tracings in patients with migraine, we must remember that from 12% to 15% of healthy people without a history of headaches, seizures, head injury or other neurological disease have EEG tracings which show non-specific abnormalities. These include excessive slow activity (at times episodic), asymmetries of the alpha rhythm, undue sensitivity to hyperventilation and occasional sharply contoured waves. Minor degrees of hypoglycaemia, changes in blood pH, medications taken by the patient, drowsiness, a family history of seizures and a variety of other factors can all cause "abnormalities" in the EEG and make it more difficult to decide if the abnormal wave forms are purely due to the patient's migraine. Only a few studies of the EEG in migraine have attempted to standardize the recording procedure and eliminate extraneous factors which could influence the tracing. Furthermore,

the opinion of electroencephalographers on the interpretation of minor abnormalities is far from uniform. Therefore, it is not surprising that the frequency
and type of abnormal EEG patterns in migraine varies considerably in the reports
published during the past 30 years.

Dow and Whitty (1947) found 59% of 51 patients with abnormal records.
In 62 sufferers from classic migraine, Heyck (1956) recorded non-specific diffuse
slow wave activity in 21% and focal abnormalities between attacks in a further
8%. Therefore, 29% of his patients had "dysrhythmic" EEG tracings. Selby and
Lance (1960) recorded EEGs from 459 of their 500 cases of migraine and allied
vascular headache. Theta (slow) activity (4Hz-7Hz) was recorded in 26% of their
patients usually in runs, and a further 3% of patients had focal slow activity in
the EEG, mainly from the temporal regions. This incidence of 29% of abnormal
EEG records increased to 40% of 74 migraineurs who suffered from impairment
of consciousness with some of their migraine attacks. The EEG tracings of two
patients contained spike and wave paroxysms; one of these patients also suffered
from epileptic seizures, but the other had neither a personal nor a family history
of epilepsy. As prominent slow activity is generally accepted as normal in the
EEG records of children, Selby and Lance (1960) eliminated children under the
age of 13 years from their calculations and found that 26% of 409 patients older
than 13 years had abnormal EEG tracings. Smyth and Winter (1964) compared
the EEG records of 202 migraine patients with a group of healthy control subjects
and recorded abnormal tracings in 43% of the migraineurs. Barolin (1969, 1971)
found 33% of abnormal EEG tracings in his patients, but the number of patients
from which this proportion was calculated was not stated. As do the authors of
several other studies, he draws attention to the excessive response to hyperventilation (53% of his patients) and to photic stimulation (11% of his cases) in
migraineurs compared with healthy control subjects. Klee (1968), who recorded
EEGs from 135 patients with a high proportion of severe migraine, found abnormal tracings in 34%. Abnormalities appeared in a further 9% only during
hyperventilation or photic stimulation. In his series, sharp waves occurred as
often as excessive slow activity. In another group of 165 patients with uncomplicated migraine, 65% of EEGs recorded in the interval between attacks were
found to contain focal or generalized slow wave abnormalities (Slatter, 1968).
The same author found an abnormal response for age to hyperventilation in only
16% of his patients; 86% of 174 migraine sufferers showed obvious following of
the cerebral rhythms to a wide range of flicker frequencies during photic stimulation, particularly with the patient's eyes open. While such a response is not
abnormal in itself, it certainly occurred in a much higher proportion of migraineurs than in the EEG tracings recorded from non-migrainous persons.

The above references were selected from an extensive literature in the hope
that averages derived from a large number of cases would eliminate some of the
variations and bias inherent in EEG recording and interpretation. The severity
of the patient's migraine, the time of obtaining the EEG after the last attack,
various extraneous factors mentioned earlier, and individual attitudes to what
is significantly abnormal in an EEG would all influence the result. Table II summarizes the findings of six papers published between 1947 and 1968. Barolin's
(1969, 1971) reports were not included because the actual number of patients
studied was not stated.

The table shows that in a total of 1024 patients with migraine, an average
of 44% had abnormal EEG results. The abnormalities were predominantly ex-

Table II. Abnormal EEG results from six papers.

Study	Number of cases	Proportion of abnormal EEG results
Dow and Whitty (1947)	51	59%
Heyck (1956)	62	29%
Selby and Lance (1960)	409 (adults)	26%
Smyth and Winter (1964)	202	43%
Klee (1968)	135	43%
Slatter (1968)	165	65%
(Total)	1024	(Average) 44%

cessive slow activity, mostly diffuse, but occasionally focal, as well as sharp waves, spikes and paroxysmal features. The latter were recorded mainly, but not exclusively, from patients who had episodes of impaired consciousness with some of their migraine attacks.

This incidence of EEG abnormalities is two to three times higher than in the non-migrainous population. Even if we allow for the fact that most of the EEGs may have been recorded from patients referred to neurologists because of unduly severe migraine, and accept that a much smaller proportion of people with common migraine seen by family physicians would have abnormal tracings, we are left in no doubt that the abnormal electrical activity of the brain in migraineurs (and, at times, in their immediate relatives) requires thought and explanation.

The extent and the type of abnormality seen in the EEGs of migraineurs recorded during headache-free periods may vary in serial tracings and, at times, may disappear. As similar abnormalities can sometimes appear in an EEG tracing of relatives who have never suffered from migraine, we must assume that the abnormal wave forms, as well as enhanced responses to hyperventilation and photic stimulation, demonstrate a disorder of cerebral function which predisposes to migraine and cannot have resulted from cerebral damage during previous migraine attacks. A similar situation applies to interseizure EEG records from epileptic patients and from some of their relatives who never had seizures. Migraine, like epilepsy, is a paroxysmal disorder of the brain, but this does not necessarily imply a direct relationship between them. In view of the fairly high frequency of persistently abnormal EEG tracings, we can propose the hypothesis that, in the majority of patients (particularly those suffering classic or complicated migraine), the primary disturbance lies somewhere in the brain and that the changes in vascular calibre, platelets, amines and synaptic transmitters are secondary to this.

The same considerations do not apply to the relatively small proportion of focal EEG changes, or to EEGs recorded during an attack of classic or complicated migraine. Here, the EEG will show a slow wave focus which may relate to appropriate visual, sensory or motor defects. In most instances, the abnormality disappears in follow-up tracings; in some, it persists permanently and indicates that ischaemic damage has occurred.

The case history of a boy with complicated migraine (described on page 86) where the CT brain scan during the attack showed marked oedema from the left frontotemporal region should be reviewed with reference to his EEG findings. The first EEG recorded during the attack showed a marked excess of bilateral 2Hz-3Hz delta activity, predominating from the left side (Fig. 6), while the results of a progress EEG recorded four weeks later were entirely normal (Fig. 8).

The range of "normality" is much wider in an EEG of a child than in that of an adult. Slow activity and various asymmetric features are physiological in the developing brain. While Bille (1962) found no essential difference in the EEG results of a large group of children with migraine compared to the tracings from a healthy control group, Prensky and Sommer (1979) recorded abnormal tracings in 73% of 64 migrainous children between 18 months and 14 years of age. About one-half of the abnormal EEGs contained excessive and diffuse slow activity, often associated with sharp waves. In 17 of these children, the EEG revealed spike, or wave and spike paroxysms; seven of these children had no personal or family history of epilepsy during follow-up periods ranging from three to nine years.

The main advantages of EEG examination are that it is non-invasive, painless, free of risk and relatively inexpensive. Apart from the interest and potential research value of recording an EEG during an attack, when should the family physician request an EEG in the routine investigation of his migraine patients? The main indications are as follow.

Indications for electroencephalography (EEG)

1. Blackouts occurring in association with the migraine attacks to assist in the decision if these are epileptic or syncopal.
2. Headaches persistently on the same side with contralateral visual, sensory or motor disorders. An EEG with focally abnormal results is a strong indication for further investigation by nuclear or computerized tomographic scanning.
3. Prolonged or persistent defects of the field of vision, or residual pareses or sensory defects.
4. A recent change in severity, duration or clinical characteristics of the migraine attack, raising a suspicion of a structural cerebral lesion.
5. Patients (even with common migraine) who have failed to respond to treatment and remain anxious about the possibility of a more serious cerebral disorder. The EEG, by providing them with further reassurance, may then be of therapeutic benefit.

It would be useful to know if an EEG, with abnormal findings recorded in the interval between attacks, provides prognostic clues for the patient's future. As yet, no studies comparing the progress of migraineurs with abnormal or normal EEG results have been published.

Other Laboratory Tests

Apart from the indications for EEG examination and for nuclear or computerized tomographic brain scans, other diagnostic procedures are required only if there are strong clinical indications for a diagnosis of "symptomatic" migraine or if there is a reasonable suspicion that ocular or sinus disease could be contributing to the patient's headaches.

Cerebral angiography should be performed only if the patient's history and results of electroencephalography and computerized tomographic brain scan are indicative of a cerebral arteriovenous malformation or tumour. It is so rare for aneurysms of intracranial arteries to cause headaches with migrainous features that this diagnosis need not be considered for practical purposes.

If the clinical criteria of a cerebral arteriovenous malformation are supported by: focal slow or sharp wave activity in the electroencephalogram on the side of hemicrania; an area of increased uptake in the nuclear scan; or a contrast enhancing lesion in the computerized tomographic brain scan, cerebral angiography is essential to demonstrate the depth and extent of the vascular malformation and its feeding and draining vessels so that the most appropriate method of treating it can be planned.

Cerebral tumours do not cause migraine or any of its variants, but a migraineur is no less likely to develop an expanding intracranial lesion than any other person. The clinical guidelines are a change in the character and duration of the patient's headaches and/or the appearance of seizures or disorders of speech, movement and sensation. The computerized tomographic brain scan can be relied on to show primary or metastatic tumours in over 90% of cases. Cerebral angiography is then needed as a preoperative examination to provide the surgeon with information about the vascularity of the mass.

Even before the advent of computerized tomographic scanning, angiography was rarely performed in the investigation of migraine. There are reports of isolated instances where the patient developed a migrainous headache during the angiographic procedure. Even then, the films did not always show the expected constriction of cerebral vessels.

Examination of the cerebrospinal fluid (CSF) has a very limited place in the investigation of migraine. It is reserved for cases where the apoplectic onset of severe headache, and neck rigidity, suggest the possibility of subarachnoid haemorrhage or meningitis. It has no value in the diagnosis of suspected tumours. The clinical presentation of intracranial bleeding and meningitis differs so much from that of migraine that the family physician should have no problem in deciding when a lumbar puncture is required.

The complex and sometimes confusing clinical features of some cases of complicated migraine (particularly in a patient's first attack) may need CSF examination to exclude a viral meningoencephalitis. In bygone days, when lumbar puncture was an integral part of neurological examination, it was clearly shown that the results of CSF examination are usually normal (both cytologically and chemically) during a migraine attack. The rare exceptions reported in the literature have not produced valid theories concerning the pathogenesis or new methods of treatment of migraine. The patient with severe complicated migraine described by Symonds (1951) and discussed on page 54 of this book, was found to have 185 neutrophils/mm^3, but there were no abnormal chemical constituents in the cerebrospinal fluid. Three days later the cell count had fallen to five neutrophils/mm^3. In a subsequent attack, with clinical features identical to the earlier ones, the CSF contained only three neutrophils/mm^3. This writer has records of a 30-year-old woman with very severe, though uncomplicated, migraine where neck rigidity motivated the family physician to perform two separate lumbar punctures six days apart. The CSF pressure was normal each time. At the first lumbar puncture, the fluid contained 200 lymphocytes/mm^3 and a raised protein level of 1.0g/L. Six days later, when the headache and neck stiffness had recovered, the CSF still contained 140 lymphocytes/mm^3, but the protein content had dropped to 0.4g/L. As neck stiffness had been a prominent feature of most of this woman's migraine attacks, and as she recovered from both headache and neck rigidity within two days, it is likely that the raised protein level and pleocytosis of her CSF were related to her migraine and not due to a benign lymphocytic meningitis.

It is generally assumed that the temporary pleocytosis and slight rise in protein content of the CSF during or just after attacks of severe migraine are due to (i) excessive permeability of small vessels allowing transudates and (ii) cerebral oedema.

Other laboratory investigations which should be considered in specific cases include the following.

Erythrocyte sedimentation rate (ESR) if the patient's age and the tenderness of the superficial temporal artery raise the possibility of giant cell (temporal) arteritis.

Measurement of *urinary catecholamine* levels to exclude phaeochromocytoma if the headaches are associated with marked rises in blood pressure.

Carotid flow studies (Doppler and scanning procedures) if prolonged focal neurological signs or a bruit heard in the neck raise the suspicion of atheroma of the cervical part of the carotid arteries in a patient with a past history of migraine.

Serum electrolyte levels should be checked, and may have to be corrected, after prolonged bouts of severe vomiting with protracted migraine attacks.

Determination of fasting *blood glucose* and *serum calcium* levels is helpful in the investigation of blackouts during or just after an attack of severe migraine, particularly if the available description of the blackout leaves the physician in doubt about its nature.

Examination by an ophthalmologist will determine *retinal vascular lesions* as a cause of persistent scotomata or other visual field defects. Intraocular pressures should be checked because the pain of glaucoma can occasionally mimic migraine. Difficulties with ocular convergence and an imbalance of eye movements can cause episodic headaches which are usually precipitated or aggravated by reading.

Examination by an ear, nose and throat surgeon is needed for a patient with no previous history of migraine when the headache is felt near the paranasal sinuses, the nose is congested, there is excessive nasal discharge and the frontal or maxillary sinuses are tender to pressure.

The number of ancillary investigations performed will vary with the experience and confidence of the primary physician. The diagnosis of migraine and of all its variants rests on taking a good history and adequate neurological examination. Ancillary investigations are needed only for differential diagnosis in the few patients with atypical clinical presentation. These will be discussed in the next chapter.

Chapter 6

Differential Diagnosis

The differential diagnosis of migraine varies with the length of the patient's history of headache, the nature of symptoms which accompany the attack, and the type of migraine variant. Therefore, a wide spectrum of conditions which could cause similar symptoms has to be considered. As the majority of patients seen by the family physician present with chronic recurring headaches, we shall proceed in our diagnostic considerations from the chronic to the subacute and finally to the first or second attack.

Chronic Recurring Headaches

Among the protean manifestations of migraine, the specific diagnostic feature is its episodic occurrence. Even though attacks of migraine may continue for several days, the patient always enjoys intervals of complete freedom from headache. This distinguishes migraine from psychogenic tension headaches where the pain continues for weeks, months or years, every day, all day, but rarely interferes with sleep. Tension headache is diffuse, and often felt in the suboccipital region, or is described as a tight band encircling the skull. It is not associated with visual symptoms before or during the headache, though some patients complain of photophobia as part of their hypersensitivity to environmental stimuli. Nausea, if it occurs, is more often caused by the large quantity of analgesic preparations consumed. Vomiting is rarely troublesome. Some patients recognize stress as the essential aggravating factor and many have other symptoms of an emotional disorder, such as insomnia, nervous dyspepsia or spastic colitis. Analgesics are consumed in vast amounts over prolonged periods, even though the patients are emphatic that they never relieve their pain. The long-held concept that chronic tension headache is caused by excessive contraction of suboccipital or scalp muscles was recently challenged. Some authors have postulated persistent extracranial vasodilatation; others have found a consistently low platelet serotonin level compared with normal control subjects. The recent interest in endorphins has stimulated a hypothesis that the patient's central mechanisms for suppressing pain perception may be deficient. It is likely that different pathogenetic mechanisms operate in individual patients; none of these theories and hypotheses has so far produced a more effective treatment of tension headaches.

Just like their non-migrainous fellows, many people with migraine are tense, anxious and unable to relax. They have to live with constant, diffuse and relatively mild headaches which hardly interrupt their work, as well as having their business and recreational activities disrupted by paroxysms of more intense migrainous pain with all the usual accompaniments. In such persons, extracranial vasodilatation may be a more important pathogenetic factor than excessive muscle contraction. A diagnosis of *tension vascular headache* has been applied to this condition. It is a useful diagnostic concept because it implies that radiological or other diagnostic investigations are only required to reassure the patient, and because it guides the physician to the most promising avenues of treatment.

An *arteriovenous malformation (AVM)* of the brain is the most important, though relatively uncommon, cause of "symptomatic" migraine. The episodic occurrence and hemicranial situation of the headache, the associated vomiting, visual and focal neurological symptoms, and the occasional good response to treatment with ergotamines may easily lead the unwary physician to a wrong diagnosis of classic migraine. In the majority of cases, but certainly not in all, the occurrence of partial (focal) seizures or the repetition of identical patterns of the visual loss (or of sensory or motor defects) will alert the physician to revise the diagnosis and to arrange appropriate investigations. The following history describes a typical case where diagnosis was delayed for many years.

A 36-year-old housewife had suffered from classic migraine since she was 10 years old. The attacks had gradually increased in frequency; in 1980, they averaged four or five a month. They were worse during the menses and, at times, were precipitated by stress. Each attack followed the same stereotyped pattern. They would begin with a visual aura of a scintillating star in the periphery of the left visual field which gradually increased in size and passed towards the centre of the visual field. This was followed by dimming of vision in the left visual field which lasted for 10 to 15 minutes. The ensuing headache was always felt around and above the right eye and in the right suboccipital region. It was extremely intense, always accompanied by photophobia and often by nausea and vomiting. The duration of headache ranged from two hours to three days with an average of four hours. Over a period of 26 years she only experienced paraesthesia of the left half of her face and of the left limbs on three occasions. During the 12 months before she was seen by the writer she had been aware of a persistent, mild defect in the lower quadrant of the left visual field. She had never lost consciousness or experienced partial seizures. Her mother and maternal grandfather had also suffered from migraine, but none of her 15 siblings did. Examination showed a slight and relative defect in the lower quadrant of the left visual field where small test objects were not seen quite as distinctly as in the upper quadrant. Movement, sensation and reflexes were normal and symmetrical. A loud bruit was heard in front of the right mastoid process, as well as on both sides of the neck, though louder on the right (the latter may have been transmitted from a benign basal systolic cardiac murmur). Prophylactic treatment with most of the commonly used preparations (including methysergide), psychotherapy and relaxation exercises had failed to reduce either the frequency or severity of her migraine. Ergotamines used at the onset of an attack, combined with analgesics, provided a measure of relief. Cerebral angiography in 1969, some 15 years after the onset of her migraine, demonstrated a huge right occipital parasagittal arteriovenous malformation supplied by both posterior cerebral arteries (Fig. 10). She was advised against surgical excision of this angioma because of its size and of the risk of causing a persistent defect of the left visual field. In 1981, branches of the right middle and posterior cerebral arteries were embolized by injection of multiple silastic emboli; subsequently, both the right and left middle meningeal and right occipital arteries were similarly embolized via catheterization of the external carotid arteries. Further angiography demonstrated that partial occlusion of the arteriovenous malformation had been achieved. At review five months later the patient reported virtual freedom from headache, but she had experienced nine transient episodes of left hemianopia, which lasted from 15 to 90 minutes.

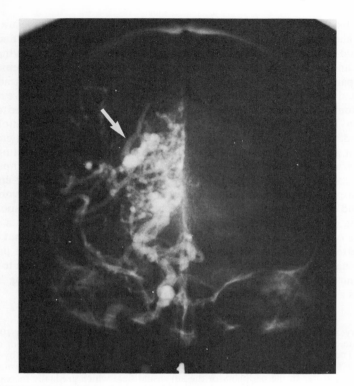

10a

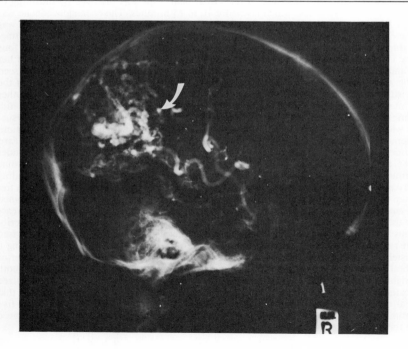

10b

This case history was recorded in some detail because it contains some of the salient features which distinguish arteriovenous malformations from classic migraine. The headaches were always right sided, while the teichopsia and hemianopia consistently involved the left visual field. The final diagnostic clue was provided by a bruit, in this case heard in front of the mastoid process, but in most cases audible over the orbits.

As many patients with a cerebral arteriovenous malformation suffer from partial (focal) or generalized seizures as well as episodic hemicranial headaches, this combination of symptoms should always arouse suspicion of the diagnosis. Subarachnoid haemorrhage arising from rupture of thin-walled vessels of the angioma is not unusual and may be the first and occasionally disastrous symptom. Other patients present with progressive intellectual impairment or with transient disorders of speech, movement or sensation caused by the stealing of blood by the angioma from other healthy regions of the brain. Depending on the nature of the clinical manifestations, some of the arteriovenous malformations may present as acute or subacute neurological problems rather than chronic recurring headaches. If the clinical picture suggests the possibility of an arteriovenous malformation, the diagnosis can now be easily confirmed or excluded by a computerized tomographic brain scan with contrast infusion or, if facilities are not available, by nuclear brain scanning.

Subacute Recurring Headache

Intracranial expanding lesions, such as abscesses, haematomas or tumours, do not usually cause episodic headaches which could be confused with migraine. Intermittent obstruction of the third or fourth ventricle, which produces an acute increase in intraventricular pressure, is the exception to this rule. This may be caused by tumours in the posterior cranial fossa which kink the cerebral aqueduct; more often, it may be caused by colloid cysts of the third ventricle. As this is one of the important neurological causes of sudden unexplained death, as abnormal neurological signs are often absent, and as they can be surgically removed, these colloid cysts must be considered in the differential diagnosis of severe migraine. The headache may be very intense, but it is generally bilateral and often precipitated by sudden changes in head posture. Vision may be blurred due to the acute and marked rise in intracranial pressure. Some patients with colloid cysts complain of brief attacks of weakness of the lower limbs which may cause them to fall to the ground without losing consciousness. The following brief case history is provided to justify the inclusion of colloid cysts of the third ventricle in the differential diagnosis of migraine.

A female medical graduate, aged 36 years, had suffered from episodic and predominantly right-sided headaches for 18 months. Some attacks were preceded by a visual aura of spots before her eyes. A neurologist had diagnosed migraine and had treated her ac-

Fig. 10. Anteroposterior and lateral projections of right carotid arteriogram showing the large right occipital parasagittal arteriovenous malformation.

cordingly. She reported that the headaches were abolished immediately by lying down, but often recurred when she sat up. This important clue, inconsistent with a diagnosis of migraine, was overlooked. After a year the headaches increased in frequency and severity progressively and were felt almost constantly across the forehead and in the nuchal region. Her memory and ability to concentrate declined and eventually brief episodes of clonic twitching of her left limbs without loss of consciousness led to her admission to hospital. She was found to have advanced bilateral papilloedema with retinal haemorrhages. Ventriculography demonstrated obliteration of the third ventricle and symmetrical dilatation of the lateral ventricles. After a shunting procedure to reduce the high intracranial pressure, the large colloid cyst was successfully removed. The patient has been well during the 11 years since this operation.

This case emphasizes the importance of a detailed history. If there is significant aggravation or rapid relief from headache by changes in posture, computerized tomographic brain scanning should be arranged long before papilloedema appears.

Giant cell (temporal) arteritis must be remembered as a cause of severe and often unilateral headache in an elderly person, even if there is a history of migraine in earlier years. The onset usually occurs after the age of 55 years; women are affected four times as frequently as men. The often intense pain may be confined to one temporal region. In contrast to migraine, this condition manifests a constant pain which interferes with sleep. A few days or weeks of general malaise and muscle pain may precede the onset of headache. Temporal arteritis is associated with polymyalgia rheumatica in about 25% of cases.

The superficial temporal artery may be palpably thickened and exquisitely tender to pressure on the painful side, but this useful diagnostic clue is absent in about 25% of cases. The erythrocyte sedimentation rate (ESR) is significantly raised, often in the vicinity of 100mm in one hour in the majority of patients. The writer believes that biopsy of the superficial temporal artery is not required if a very high ESR supports the clinical diagnosis. In almost 30% of patients with giant cell arteritis, the ESR may be only 40mm in one hour or even less. Biopsy is then essential. A long segment of the artery must be examined as the arteritic process may skip segments of the arterial wall. As the disease involves the ophthalmic, vertebral and other intracranial arteries, as well as the superficial temporal artery, early diagnosis and treatment are essential to prevent the risk of severe and irreversible visual impairment and, less commonly, cerebral infarction. Corticosteroid therapy is usually effective in abolishing headache and in preventing complications. The dose of corticosteroids and the necessity to continue treatment, often for several years, are determined from the ESR.

There are a few other conditions which should be considered as a cause of episodic severe pain in the head, either generalized or unilateral. These include:

Sudden paroxysmal sharp *rises in blood pressure,* which cause an acute, generalized "explosive" headache similar to that of subarachnoid haemorrhage. This may occur in people taking monoamine oxidase inhibitor drugs for a depressive illness and who have ingested tyramine-containing foods. If the patient has not taken such drugs or foods, repeated estimations of urinary catecholamine levels and other appropriate tests are required to exclude a phaeochromocytoma.

Acute or subacute frontal *sinusitis* and *neoplasms of the paranasal sinuses.* Though often constant, the pain may remit. Tenderness over the frontal sinuses, malaise, fever, and nasal congestion are indications. X-ray examinations of the paranasal sinuses will establish the correct diagnosis.

Angle-closure *glaucoma* may present with intermittent, severe periorbital pain and blurring of vision. This may lead to an erroneous impression of migraine. The history is

Table III. Differential diagnosis of subacute or chronic recurring headache

Diagnosis	Site	Aggravating factors	Nausea and/ or vomiting	Visual disorders	Focal cerebral symptoms	Laboratory investigations	Diagnostic clues
Migraine	Hemicranial or bilateral	Multiple	+ or −	Photophobia ? visual aura	Sensory or motor ipsilateral with hemicrania	None specific	See text
Tension headache	Frontal or suboccipital	Stress	Usually −	−	−	−	Anxious personality, little relief from analgesics
Arteriovenous malformation	Often hemicranial	−	+ or −	Hemianopia contralateral to hemicrania	−	CT brain scan Angiography	Focal seizures, bruits in 50% of cases
Intermittent hydrocephalus	Generalized	Change in head posture	+ or −	Transient blurring	−	Large ventricles in CT brain scan	Progressive history → papilloedema
Temporal arteritis	Hemicranial or bilateral	−	−	Occasional	−	High ESR, temporal artery biopsy	Over age 55 years, polymyalgia rheumatica
Paroxysmal hypertension	Bilateral	Tyramine-containing foods in patients taking MAO inhibitors	+ or −	−	−	Urinary catecholamines, CT scan of adrenals	Severe hypertension during headache
Angle closure glaucoma	Periorbital or generalized	−	−	+	−	Tonometry	Blurring of vision persists

subacute; autonomic and other accompanying features of a migraine attack are absent. The visual blurring lasts longer than is usual in vascular headache. Persistent visual loss can be avoided by early referral to an ophthalmologist who will make the correct diagnosis and supervise treatment with the aid of tonometry.

Acute Headache

When the primary physician is summoned to see the patient during the first attack of overwhelming headache, a diagnosis of migraine can be made only from characteristic visual prodromata and from a hemicranial situation of pain. Photophobia and vomiting occur in meningitis and viral meningoencephalitis as much as in migraine. Focal cerebral disorders are more likely to result from encephalitis or subarachnoid haemorrhage than from migraine. Pyrexia is not invariable at the onset of a viral encephalitis and is relatively uncommon in subarachnoid bleeding. In both conditions, neck rigidity and demonstration of a positive Kernig's sign may appear only after a few hours. Small subarachnoid leaks, which stop spontaneously and may recur after days or weeks, are a treacherous, but rare, pitfall in diagnosis. In such cases, particularly if neck rigidity is present, the cerebrospinal fluid should be examined to determine whether the cause is bacterial or viral meningitis or subarachnoid bleeding. However, we have records of a number of patients (mostly younger than 30 years) with a clinical presentation characteristic of viral meningitis, including headache and photophobia for several days, where the cerebrospinal fluid contained no excess of cells and the chemical composition of the fluid remained normal.

Cluster Headache

Many patients with cluster headaches who have been referred to a neurologist have previously been wrongly diagnosed and unsuccessfully treated for trigeminal and other facial neuralgias. The clinical features of these conditions are so characteristic that correct diagnosis should present no difficulty. In trigeminal neuralgia, the paroxysms of pain are usually triggered by eating, talking or touching the face; they rarely occur at night and they are not accompanied by lacrimation or congestion of the nostril. The pain is felt over one or more divisions of the trigeminal nerve. The eye and forehead (ophthalmic division) are often spared. The pain of "atypical facial neuralgia" is mostly constant, often bilateral, and rarely extends into the forehead. It is never accompanied by a running eye or nose.

In contrast, cluster headache occurs in well defined bouts during which from one to four attacks appear in 24 hours. Often, one of these is nocturnal. The pain is not triggered by any environmental circumstances or manoeuvres. It is usually accompanied by watering of the eye and congestion of the nose on the side of pain. The clinical characteristics of cluster headache and of its chronic variant were described in detail in Chapter 4.

Lower Half Headache

This uncommon migraine variant should not be difficult to distinguish from trigeminal or atypical facial neuralgia and from pain due to temporomandibular

Table IV. Differential diagnosis of acute headache

Diagnosis	Site	Neck rigidity	Nausea and/or vomiting	Visual disorders	Focal cerebral symptoms	Laboratory investigations
First attack of migraine	Hemicranial or bilateral	–	+ or –	+ or –	+ or –	Negative
Encephalitis or meningitis	Suboccipital or generalized	+	+	Photophobia	+ or –	CSF pleocytosis
Subarachnoid haemorrhage	Suboccipital or generalized	+	+	– or ocular palsies	+ or –	CSF blood-stained and xanthochromic
Subdural haematoma	Focal or generalized	–	+ or –	– but ? unequal pupils	+ or –	CT brain scan

joint dysfunction (Costen's syndrome). Lower half headache can be bilateral or alternating from side to side. Many patients report an antecedent or concurrent history of more conventional migraine and photophobia, nausea and vomiting, as well as the long duration of pain. The absence of specific trigger factors are clinical criteria against a diagnosis of facial neuralgia.

In temporomandibular joint dysfunction, pain is usually confined to one side, but it may be bilateral. It is episodic, lasting minutes or hours, and is sometimes precipitated by eating. It may radiate over most of the face and into the neck. Tenderness to pressure over the temporomandibular joint and an irregular bite are diagnostic clues which require the patient's referral to a dental surgeon interested and experienced in the treatment of dental malocclusion.

Chronic Paroxysmal Hemicrania

The chronic form of cluster headache, which Pearce (1980) called "chronic migrainous neuralgia", must now be distinguished from a rare headache entity described by Sjaastad and Dale in 1974 and later called "chronic paroxysmal hemicrania". To date, less than 10 cases of this condition have been reported in the literature. Only one of these had a preceding history of typical cluster headache — this had responded to treatment with ergotamine. In contrast to either the typical or chronic form of cluster headache, patients with chronic paroxysmal hemicrania experience from four to twelve attacks of pain each day for years without remission. The pain is centred around the eye and radiates to the temple or cheek. Each attack lasts from five to 60 minutes and, contrary to cluster headache, nocturnal pain is unusual. Headache consistently remains on the same side and may be associated with conjunctival congestion and a clear discharge from the nostril on this side. Treatment with ergotamines, methysergide, pizotifen, corticosteroids and carbamazepine is not effective, but the outstanding and remarkable clinical feature is an almost immediate and complete abolition of pain by the administration of indomethacin. Hemicrania recurs only if this treatment is interrupted.

The writer has elected not to include chronic paroxysmal hemicrania in the description of migraine and its variants because its pathogenesis is uncertain and the specific and dramatic response to treatment with indomethacin does not apply to any other migraine variant. It may have a vascular component — indomethacin is known to have some constrictive effect on cranial vessels. Indomethacin (as well as aspirin, which was reported to diminish the pain of chronic paroxysmal hemicrania) is known to inhibit prostaglandin synthesis. The pathogenesis of this very rare headache entity may depend more on mechanisms involving vasoactive prostaglandins than any of the more common variants of the migraine syndrome. The importance of considering chronic paroxysmal hemicrania in the differential diagnosis of migraine and cluster headache lies in the potential for complete success from treatment with indomethacin.

Migraine without Headache

Visual Symptoms

In Chapter 4 it was mentioned (page 58) that transient visual symptoms such as shimmering crescents and scotomas can occur without ensuing headache

Table V. Differential diagnosis of cluster headache

Diagnosis	Site	Frequency	Triggers	Lacrimation	Duration	Diagnostic clues
Cluster headache	Strictly hemicranial supraorbital	Up to 6 attacks in 24 hours during cluster	—	+	30–90 mins.	Clusters
Trigeminal neuralgia	1, 2 or all 3 divisions of trigeminal nerve on same side	Several daily	Talking, chewing, touching face	—	Seconds or minutes, repetitive	Remissions
Atypical facial neuralgia	Unilateral or bilateral	Constant	Stress	—	Usually constant	Tense personality
Lower half headache	Hemicranial or bilateral	Episodic	—	—	Hours	Past history of migraine
Temporomandibular joint dysfunction	Uni- or bilateral radiates to neck	Episodic, no remissions	Chewing, yawning	—	Minutes to hours	Malocclusion of bite

or nausea. If the patient recalls a preceding history of classic or common migraine, the diagnosis should be obvious. The diagnosis becomes more difficult if a person with such visual disturbances has never suffered from vascular headaches and is not aware of a family history of migraine. An intelligent and observant person may be able to describe or draw the scintillating crescent, often with a serrated edge. The crescent tends to travel from the periphery to the centre of the visual field of one eye and is often followed by a partial scotoma. In such cases, any doubt of a retinal vascular lesion should be resolved by ophthalmological examination. If the patient experiences only transient and diffuse visual blurring, without a scintillating scotoma, stenosis or atheroma of the internal carotid artery must be considered. This diagnosis becomes more obvious (i) if some of the episodes of visual loss in one eye are associated with temporary weakness or paraesthesia in the contralateral limbs; (ii) if a bruit is heard over the carotid artery in the neck; or (iii) if small platelet or cholesterol emboli can be discovered in branches of the retinal artery. Carotid flow studies, including Echo flow, should then be performed before deciding on the necessity for cerebral angiography.

Recurrent brief episodes of monocular blindness (amaurosis fugax) may also occur in the absence of a source or signs of retinal arterial embolism. The visual impairment comes on gradually and progresses from dimming to complete blindness; recovery similarly proceeds in a gradual fashion. The duration of blindness is from a few seconds to 30 minutes, with an average of from two to five minutes. There are no visual hallucinations and no pain is felt around the eye or in the head. Recovery is complete and, as yet, no permanent visual defect has been reported. In a series of 12 patients with this condition reported by Eadie, Sutherland and Tyrer (1968), the mean age of the patients was 29.5 years. Only one was over 40 years old. Carotid angiography was performed in eight patients, but no abnormality was demonstrated. The recurrent blindness usually affects the same eye, but may alternate from eye to eye. As it is monocular, the causative lesion must be in the retina or optic nerve. The short duration and subsequent complete recovery are consistent with retinal angiospasm, but this has not been proven. The absence of scintillating and migrating scotomas distinguishes this recurrent monocular blindness from visual migraine without headache which is also presumed to be caused by spasm of the retinal arteries.

Vertigo

A sense of rotation of the patient or of the environment is experienced as an aura by a proportion of people with classic migraine. The feeling usually continues for two to five minutes. It is accompanied by ataxia, but not by aural discomfort or tinnitus. Such vertigo and ataxia may occur without subsequent headache or nausea, particularly in post-menopausal women who had suffered from migraine before the menopause. The pathogenesis is assumed to include reduced perfusion through the labyrinthine end arteries. This would be in agreement with the occurrence of transient visual, sensory or motor defects in migrainous subjects without headache.

The diagnosis of migrainous angiospastic vertigo rests on a preceding history of migraine and on the short duration of giddiness (usually less than five minutes and rarely exceeding 20 minutes). The absence of aural discomfort, deafness and tinnitus distinguishes it from recurrent labyrinthine vertigo (Meniere's syndrome). Transient vertebrobasilar ischaemia should be considered in the differential diagnosis, but in this condition the feeling of giddinesss is more prolonged. Some of the recurrent episodes may be accompanied by dysarthria, diplopia or other symptoms of brain stem ischaemia. Auscultation for a bruit arising from the origin of the vertebral artery in the supraclavicular region should always be performed.

More detailed descriptions and case histories of patients with migrainous vertigo and without headache can be found in Chapter 4 (pages 44-46).

Transient Disorders of Speech, Movement and Sensation

In previous chapters of this book it was mentioned that temporary disorders of speech, movement and sensation often occur either as an aura or during an attack of classic migraine. Whereas retinal or vestibular migrainous angiospasm without headache is not unusual, the same does not apply to focal cerebral disorders. On occasions, subjects with a past history of classic migraine may experience numbness or paraesthesia of one side of the face or a hand without headache. However, migrainous dysphasia or hemiparesis rarely occurs without headache. Therefore, transient carotid ischaemia is a more likely diagnosis in a patient presenting with focal cerebral disorders without headache, even if such a patient has a personal past history or a family history of classic migraine. It should not be forgotten that unilateral, often frontal or periorbital headache, occurs occasionally in embolic or thrombotic focal cerebral ischaemia. The discovery of subtle, mild objective sensory defects, a drift of the outstretched arm, exaggerated tendon reflexes on the previously paretic side, or an arterial bruit in the neck support the necessity for further investigation. This includes elimination of risk factors (arteritis, polycythaemia, hyperlipidaemia) and studies of carotid blood flow by all the available methods. If a bruit is heard, and if the flow studies reveal a significant abnormality, angiographic demonstration of the cervical parts of the carotid and vertebral arteries will assist the decision for endarterectomy or other vascular surgical procedures to reduce the risk of recurrence.

Ocular Palsies

Ophthalmoplegic migraine, though uncommon, can cause considerable diagnostic problems, particularly if the patient is seen during the first attack. The oculomotor (third) nerve is selectively involved in 90% of cases, but either an abducens or a trochlear palsy can occur in isolation. Some patients present with a complete ophthalmoplegia. The diagnosis of ophthalmoplegic migraine becomes likely if: (i) the patient has a past history of common or classic migraine; (ii) headache precedes the painful ocular palsy; and (iii) the ophthalmoplegia persists for some time after the headache has subsided. The occurrence of previous attacks of ocular muscle paralysis on the same or opposite side strongly indicates a migrainous aetiology. Chapter 4 (pages 49-50) contains a more detailed account of ophthalmoplegic migraine.

If the patient is seen during the first attack and there is any doubt about the migrainous nature of the ocular palsy, an unruptured aneurysm of the circle of Willis must be excluded by both carotid and vertebral angiography. Diabetes has to be considered as a cause of ocular muscle palsies. Appropriate investigations should be performed to exclude the more remote possibilities of syphilis, endocrine ophthalmopathy and orbital mucocele. Myasthenia gravis can cause recurrent and fluctuating ptosis and partial ocular muscle pareses. The immediate clinical distinction from ophthalmoplegic migraine is the absence of pain and sparing of the pupil in myasthenia gravis.

Migraine Syncope

The distinction between syncope and epilepsy as a cause of a "blackout" during attacks of migraine may be difficult. If the description by the patient or by witnesses does not provide clear diagnostic data, electroencephalography should be performed, bearing in mind that normal interictal electroencephalography does not exclude epilepsy. The border between severe syncope and epilepsy is not sharply defined. As a general rule, syncope is more likely than epilepsy during an attack of migraine. Incontinence may occur in both conditions if the bladder happens to be full when the patient loses consciousness. Anticonvulsant treatment should be prescribed only after more than one blackout and if the clinical features or electroencephalographic findings favour epilepsy.

Chapter 7

Treatment

Migraine and its many variants are episodic, recurrent diseases which may persist throughout the patient's life. No complete cure is known at present. Therapeutic efforts are directed at reducing the frequency and duration of attacks and at alleviating pain and associated symptoms once an attack occurs. Once consideration has been given to the multiplicity of factors, including the patient's personality and emotional make-up, and the many environmental triggers which contribute to the genesis of common migraine, several avenues of prophylaxis may have to be explored and tailored to the needs of the individual migrainous person.

Prevention

In general, the frequency of attacks is higher in common migraine than in the classic and complicated forms of the disease and in most variants. The patient's personality structure, emotional state and environmental circumstances are much more important in common migraine than in the classic and other forms of migraine. Therefore, the scope for prevention and the potential for therapeutic success is greatest in common migraine. Prophylaxis may be achieved by pharmacological and non-pharmacological methods. However, the latter have only limited value in the management of a patient with classic or complicated migraine.

Drug Treatment

Controlled trials and many years of clinical experience have shown that a number of drugs are capable of reducing the frequency and severity of migraine in up to 60% of patients. Complete prevention is rarely achieved, but it is not unrealistic to aim for a 50% to 75% reduction in the number of attacks. As all drugs have side effects — usually minor, but often elaborated by the patient — they should be prescribed only for persons who suffer an average of more than one attack per month. This high frequency is unusual in classic migraine and very rare in all forms of complicated migraine. The drug of first choice should be determined from the individual characteristics of the patient, but it may be necessary to try several drugs before the one which suits a particular person, and has least side effects, is found.

We shall describe the therapeutic and the potential adverse effects of each of the drugs currently used for the prevention of migraine. We shall also mention their interactions with other drugs, pharmacological data, contraindications, and provide some guidelines for their use in specific patients. During the past 50 years, a multitude of remedies has been claimed to prevent migraine. Until recently, none had been subjected to controlled trials. In an episodic disease as complex and variable as common migraine and where the frequency of attacks depends on many and heterogeneous factors, clinical trials testing the effect of a drug for less than six months, or even less than twelve months, must be interpreted with caution. The patient's anticipation of relief from a "new" drug increases the chance of success, at least initially. Many clinical trials have shown that from 35% to 40% of patients obtain marked relief from the placebo drug compared with 50% of migraineurs who responded to the active drug in the trial.

Although the physiological and biochemical events which contribute to the pathogenesis of migraine are not well understood and remain subject to controversy, the interval prophylactic treatment of migraine employs pharmaceutical preparations which either: (i) tend to enhance the vasoconstrictor tone of extracranial arteries; or (ii) alter serotonin action.

1. Drugs which enhance constriction of extracranial arteries

A. Ergotamine. This alkaloid of ergot has been used for the treatment of migraine since 1925 (Fanchamps, 1976). As it is employed more widely for the treatment of an attack of migraine headache than for prevention, the pharmacology and toxicity of ergotamine will be described later in this chapter. If vascular tone is low, ergotamine in therapeutic doses causes peripheral vasoconstriction mainly by stimulating alpha-adrenergic receptors. It is also an antagonist of serotonin and reduces the increased rate of platelet aggregation induced by serotonin (American Hospital Formulary Service, 1981).

The widespread constriction of peripheral arteries precludes the prolonged use of ergotamine in large doses for the prevention of migraine. However, it may be prescribed intermittently for patients who suffer migraine attacks: (i) mainly at weekends; (ii) in association with menstruation; (iii) for the prevention of an attack following an anticipated stress situation. In these circumstances the oral administration of 1mg to 2mg ergotamine tartrate at night, or twice daily for two to three days, may protect the patient from a vascular headache.

Bellergal, a compound preparation containing 0.3mg of ergotamine tartrate, 0.1mg of belladonna alkaloids and 20mg of phenobarbitone, has been prescribed for the prevention of migraine and symptoms of vasomotor instability for well over 30 years. The average dose is one tablet, three times daily. Lance (1972b) found Bellergal effective in about 35% of patients. Although such small doses of ergotamine will result in only low serum levels of the drug, and although current medical thought will be dismayed about the long-term use of even small doses of phenobarbitone, the writer has prescribed Bellergal for hundreds of patients during the past 30 years. The drug should be considered for persons suffering from common migraine where emotional tension precipitates attacks — and particularly for those patients who also complain of frequent vasomotor dizziness and syncope. The author has not yet seen or heard of a patient who developed signs of ergotism or who became dependent on Bellergal even after years of regular use. Drowsiness is the main side effect, possibly requiring reduction in dose or withdrawal of the drug. Rashes, presumably due to the barbiturate, and nausea occur infrequently and recover rapidly once the drug is withdrawn. Bellergal is also available in a "retard" formulation which contains twice the amount of each of the three ingredients of the ordinary Bellergal tablet. If taken before going to bed, this dosage is useful for the prevention of vascular headaches beginning during sleep or in the early morning hours. As the 40mg phenobarbitone contained in a Bellergal Retard tablet may cause drowsiness, many patients do not like taking it in the morning. The cost of both formulations of Bellergal tablets is fairly high and patients should be advised of this before it is prescribed.

B. Clonidine. This drug is an alpha-adrenergic agonist, but it also has alpha-adrenergic blocking activity. It is an imidazoline derivative, used in higher dosage for the treatment of hypertension and in a small dose (averaging 75µg per day) for the prophylaxis of migraine. The vasoconstrictive action of clonidine is assumed to be due to alpha-adrenergic stimulation. Observations on its success in the prophylaxis of migraine in relatively small series of patients for periods of up to 12 months were conflicting (Heathfield and Raiman, 1972; Shaw and Saunders, 1972). The writer has a very limited experience with clonidine because the patients treated with it initially failed to respond. However, Tallett (1972), points out that a significant response may appear only after weeks or months of therapy.

No information is available on the interaction of other drugs with the small doses of clonidine used for the prophylaxis of migraine. Common side effects include drowsiness and a dry mouth; nausea, vomiting, agitation, depression, palpitations, faintness and hypotension have also been recorded (Eadie and Tyrer, 1980).

From discussions with other neurologists and with family physicians, and from the dearth of literature in recent years, it would appear that clonidine reduces the frequency and severity of migraine in an occasional patient. However, it appears to have no specific advantages over other drugs used for prophylaxis.

C. Propranolol. Clinical trials of some beta-adrenergic blocking drugs, including pindolol, alprenolol and oxprenolol, showed that they were no more effective than a placebo in preventing migraine attacks. Although beta-receptors have been identified in both cerebral and extracranial vessels, and the simple hypothesis that beta-blockers can prevent spasm of intracranial vessels and dilation of extracranial arteries seemed attractive, it is unlikely that beta-blockade has any significant effect on the course of migraine.

However, propranolol was found to be effective in the prophylaxis of migraine. Several controlled clinical trials with a total of nearly 250 patients, followed up for periods ranging from three to 24 months, reported a better than 50% reduction in the frequency and severity of migraine attacks in from 55% to 93% of patients treated with propranolol (Widerøe and Vigander, 1974; Diamond and Medina, 1976). Beta-blockade is unlikely to be responsible for this good therapeutic effect, but an antagonism of propranolol to both noradrenaline and serotonin has been demonstrated. Although the mechanism of action of the drug is not clearly understood, it is thought to block the dilation of cranial arteries and arterioles caused by low concentrations of serotonin (Raskin, 1981).

The recommended daily dose of propranolol in adults ranges from 80mg to 160mg. Treatment should be started with 40mg twice daily and increased gradually, if necessary, up to 40mg four times daily. For children over the age of seven years, treatment should be started with 10mg once or twice daily and increased slowly, as required, up to 2mg/kg body weight per day in divided doses.

The prophylactic effect of propranolol may be slow to appear; a trial of this drug should be continued for at least three months.

The plasma half-life of orally administered propranolol is two to five hours, but the therapeutic effect lasts for about 10 hours. It is metabolized primarily by the liver. Propranolol produces bradycardia and decreased cardiac output and may cause a degree of bronchospasm. It enhances the actions of some anti-hypertensive drugs and increases the effects of insulin and orally administered hypoglycaemic agents. Therefore, it should not be prescribed for persons with a history of asthma or chronic obstructive airways disease. Special caution is needed for patients with a past history of impaired myocardial function and for diabetics. As the drug is used widely as an antihypertensive it should be the first choice for migraineurs where high blood pressure may have contributed to an increased frequency or severity of headaches. Propranolol is known to have anxiolytic properties, possibly through its antagonism of noradrenaline. Therefore it should be considered for anxious patients in whom exposure to even minor stress may precipitate a migraine attack.

Side effects are reported by no more than 5% to 10% of patients taking propranolol in the doses recommended for migraine prophylaxis. Side effects include dizziness, presumably due to hypotension and insomnia. More often they consist of vivid dreams, nightmares or hallucinations. On rare occasions, propranolol may cause drowsiness and depression. Rashes, purpura and fever were reported as idiosyncratic toxic effects (Eadie and Tyrer, 1980). Although there are no data on human dysmorphogenicity, propranolol, like most other drugs, should not be used during pregnancy.

In the writer's experience, migraine prophylaxis with propranolol was not as successful as the results of controlled clinical trials had promised. This may be due to a lower dose of propranolol, averaging about 120mg per day, or to the fact that a number of patients discontinued the drug after only four to eight weeks if further attacks of migraine occurred. However, on a few occasions migraine headaches ceased completely, even though adequate treatment with various other drugs had failed. It seems possible that there is a subgroup of migraineurs with specific pathogenetic mechanisms which respond better to propranolol than to other drugs available for migraine prophylaxis.

Although reports of single cases cannot be accepted as evidence for the value of any drug in the prevention of an illness as complex as migraine, the following spectacular therapeutic success convinced the writer that treatment with propranolol merits a trial.

A 13-year-old schoolgirl with a past history of only three attacks of migraine since the age of 10 years, began to experience three to four attacks of severe classic migraine each month, unrelated to any apparent triggers in her environment. The aura consisted of blurring or of complete loss of vision, of hemianopic defects of the visual field or of patchy scotomata. Vision recovered after 10 minutes, but a severe headache followed at first confined to the right side and later spreading to the left. Photophobia and nausea occurred in all attacks. Occasionally, she vomited. She would then lie down in a quiet room and sleep. She felt well, but tired, on waking. Results of electroencephalography and a nuclear brain scan showed no significant abnormality. Attempts at prophylactic treatment with ergotamine (Bellergal), pizotifen and methysergide over a period of four months completely failed to prevent her migraine. Propranolol was then introduced in a 10mg dose twice daily and the attacks ceased completely. After six months the dose of propranolol was reduced to 5mg twice daily. Migraine did not recur unless the patient forgot to take at least two doses of the drug. She has remained well for three years after starting treatment with such a small dose of propranolol.

In summary, propranolol can be safely prescribed for migraine prophylaxis and has fewer side effects than some of the other drugs in current use. About 50% of patients can be expected to respond favourably to the drug, particularly those in whom anxiety or hypertension contribute to vascular headaches of migraine type. Propranolol should not be used for patients with asthma and chronic bronchitis and special care is needed when offering it to diabetics or to patients with congestive cardiac failure.

2. Drugs which alter serotonin action

Serotonin is widely regarded as the most important vasoactive amine involved in the pathogenesis of migraine. When plasma serotonin levels were found to fall during a migraine headache (Curran, Hinterberger and Lance, 1965), the antiserotonin action of some drugs failed to provide a satisfactory explanation for their success in migraine prophylaxis. It was then proposed that methysergide, a serotonin antagonist, may occupy receptor sites on the arterial wall and so block the vascular responses to fluctuations in levels of plasma serotonin. Another theory is concerned more with brain serotonin which is contained within specific neural circuits. Some originate from cell bodies located in the mid-brain raphe nuclei. Fibres containing serotonin were shown to pass from these nuclei to cortical parenchymal microvessels (Törk, 1982). The so-called serotonin "antagonists" actually mimic the action of serotonin within the central nervous system by depressing the firing rate of central raphe neurons. They are therefore serotonin agonists and not antagonists in the serotonergic circuits in the brain. Raskin (1981) suggests that a defect in the modulation of transmitter release, resulting in intermittently low synaptic serotonin levels, may be involved in the pathogenesis of migraine. He also suggests that the common mode of action of agents effective for prevention could be a depression of the firing rate of mid-brain serotonergic neurons.

As mentioned above, propranolol might be included among the drugs which alter serotonin action. It appears to be an inhibitor of the uptake of serotonin by platelets. It may also block the dilation of cranial arterioles caused by low concentrations of serotonin (Raskin, 1981).

Three drugs which have both antiserotonin and antihistaminic actions are widely used for migraine prevention. The chemical structures of these drugs show some similarities.

A. Cyproheptadine. This drug is more often prescribed as an antihistamine than for migraine prophylaxis. It is also a peripheral serotonin antagonist, but it has less vasoactivity than methysergide. It does not block the vasoconstrictor action of serotonin in branches of the carotid artery. Cyproheptadine has weak anticholinergic and antibradykinin activity. It is said to prevent platelet aggregation. This may contribute to its therapeutic effect in the prevention of migraine (Raskin, 1981).

As drowsiness is a common side effect of cyropheptadine, it is advisable to prescribe it in a 4mg dose at night only. Some patients will tolerate 4mg twice daily, but few will be able to take larger doses without feeling sleepy. Sedatives, including alcohol, enhance the soporific effect of the drug. Cyproheptadine increases appetite, consequently causing weight gain. Therefore many patients, particularly women, refuse to persevere with it. Other dose-related toxicity includes a dry mouth and dizziness.

B. Methdilazine. This drug has similar properties to cyproheptadine, but probably causes less weight gain. The side effect of drowsiness again limits its use. Doses higher than 4mg to 8mg at night, or twice daily, are rarely tolerated. In the writer's experience, neither cyproheptadine nor methdilazine was found to be highly effective for prevention of migraine. Their use is recommended mainly for patients who suffer from allergic disorders, such as rhinitis, in addition to migraine. They should be tried if other drugs are not effective or produce intolerable side effects.

C. Pizotifen. This drug is an antagonist of serotonin and histamine and also has weak anticholinergic and antibradykinin properties. Spontaneous platelet aggregation, abnormally high in the majority of migraine patients, is significantly reduced by pizotifen (Mazal and Rachmilewitz, 1980). The drug became available for clinical trial in 1966, shortly after the uncommon, but serious, side effects of methysergide had been reported. It does not directly constrict the vessel wall, nor does it potentiate the vasoconstrictor action of serotonin or noradrenaline.

The results of controlled clinical trials have shown a significant reduction in the frequency and severity of migraine in from 50% to 70% of patients treated with pizotifen (Sicuteri *et al.,*, 1967; Lance *et al.,* 1970). In an open clinical trial of 27 patients with common migraine and 11 patients with classic migraine of whom 42.5% were treated for longer than six months, treatment with pizotifen was found to be more effective in the management of classic than of common migraine. Only two patients reported complete freedom from headache, but the incidence or severity of attacks was significantly reduced in a further 55% of cases (Selby, 1970).

Pizotifen appears to have less sedative effect than either cyproheptadine or methdilazine. It has some antidepressant properties which may be useful in treating the depressed migraineur. Its plasma half-life is from 22 to 26 hours. Therefore, administration in the morning and evening should suffice, although no adequate data are available on plasma level correlations (Eadie and Tyrer, 1980). It is available in tablets containing 0.5mg (base).

Drowsiness may be avoided by starting treatment with 0.5mg pizotifen at night and by increasing the dose gradually by an additional 0.5mg tablet at intervals of one week, to reach a daily dose ranging from 1.0mg to 2.5mg.

Drowsiness and fatigue tend to limit the dose, but the most common and important side effect is weight gain, which is unacceptable to many female patients. If most migraine attacks occur in association with the menstrual cycle or with specific environmental circumstances, the intermittent administration of pizotifen for no longer than two weeks each month may reduce the increase in weight and enable some patients to persevere with the drug. Dizziness and nausea are minor and uncommon side effects.

Although pizotifen is not as effective as methysergide, the absence of serious side effects makes it a drug of first choice for patients who experience vascular headaches more often than once or twice a month. Its antidepressant and sedative properties favour its use for the treatment of persons who suffer from both tension headaches and migraine.

D. Methysergide. Methysergide is the most effective drug for the prevention of severe migraine, but its use is limited by the infrequent occurrence of potentially serious side effects. It is a lysergic acid derivative with some structural resemblance to ergotamine.

The mechanism of action of methysergide in the prophylaxis of migraine is not known. It is a competitive serotonin antagonist peripherally, but it may act as a serotonin agonist centrally on the serotonergic pathways arising in the midbrain. It inhibits histamine release by mast cells, reduces release of serotonin from platelets, and blocks the effects of serotonin on receptors; thereby, it may reduce the permeability of small blood vessels. It is possible, but difficult to prove, that the success of methysergide in migraine prophylaxis is due more to its central serotonin agonist effect than to its peripheral serotonin antagonism.

The first results from clinical trials with methysergide were published in 1959. Bruyn and Gathier (1968) collated the reports of various authors and concluded that methysergide was effective in preventing vascular headache of migraine type in some 70% of over 2700 patients. Lance (1972b) found that regular medication with methysergide in a dose of from 2mg to 6mg per day suppresses migraine completely in about 20% of patients and achieves a substantial improvement in a further 45% of cases. The beneficial effects do not decline even after years of treatment. However, treatment must be interrupted for three to four weeks every four to six months to prevent the rare side effect of retroperitoneal, pleural or cardiac valvular fibrosis.

The high success rate of methysergide in the prevention of migraine is offset by a fairly high incidence of relatively minor side effects, particularly during the early weeks of therapy. Up to 40% of patients complained of nausea, abdominal cramps, anorexia, diarrhoea and, rarely, vomiting. Some feel drowsy, dizzy or faint; a few become euphoric. Hallucinations were reported in isolated instances. Various other psychic disturbances, such as difficulty with thinking, feelings of depersonalization and reactions similar to those which occur with the use of lysergic acid diethylamide (LSD) have occurred mainly after high doses of methysergide. More important, but not unduly frequent, are the vasoconstrictor effects of the drug which can cause pain, pallor and coldness of the extremities. There have been rare reports of claudication of the legs and angina pectoris. Loss of scalp hair has also been reported, but this may abate even if treatment with methysergide is continued.

Connective tissue disorders, including retroperitoneal fibrosis and, less often, pleural and cardiac valvular fibrosis, have developed after long-term uninterrupted administration of methysergide. Graham (1967) found reports of such connective tissue diseases in about 100 of an estimated 500 000 people who had been treated with methysergide. Lance (1972b) had seen one case of chronic pleural fibrosis and one of retroperitoneal fibrosis among 1000 patients treated with the drug for up to six years. It is now known that these connective tissue reactions can be prevented by interrupting the administration of methysergide for four weeks every four to six months. It was also found that symptoms of these fibrotic syndromes resolve within a few weeks after withdrawal of the drug.

The common gastrointestinal and other minor side effects (such as dizziness, lethargy or insomnia) can often be prevented by introducing methysergide in a 1mg dose at night and by gradual 1mg increments at weekly intervals. Nausea and abdominal cramps can be reduced by taking the drug immediately after meals. Often, the early side effects disappear after a few weeks, but about 10%

of patients cannot tolerate methysergide either because of the persistence of un-pleasant symptoms or because they experience precordial pain or manifesta-tions of peripheral vasoconstriction in their extremities. These symptoms are reversible when treatment with the drug is discontinued. Rebound headache, which may occur on abrupt withdrawal of the drug, can be prevented by reducing the dose gradually over two to three weeks.

Methysergide is contraindicated in patients with: (i) ischaemic heart disease; (ii) severe hypertension; (iii) atherosclerosis (particularly peripheral vascular dis-ease); (iv) phlebitis of the lower limbs; (v) peptic ulcer; (vi) impaired hepatic or renal function; (vii) valvular heart disease; or (viii) a history of collagen diseases. Although there is no definite evidence of dysmorphogenicity, the drug should not be prescribed during pregnancy. The vasoconstrictor effect of methysergide may be enhanced by ergotamines and by sympathomimetic agents.

The drug is marketed in Australia and in the United Kingdom in tablets containing 1mg methysergide. In the USA, each tablet contains 2mg methyser-gide maleate.

The average dose ranges from 2mg to 6mg per day. As the half-life of the drug in man is only about two hours, and as peak plasma levels are reached about two hours after administration (Eadie and Tyrer, 1980), methysergide should be taken three times daily. However, it is advisable to start treatment with 1mg at night and to increase the dose gradually by 1mg each week to avoid side effects. If the drug does not prevent the patient's migraine after four weeks on an adequate dose, it should be withdrawn.

The high incidence of side effects implies that methysergide is not the drug of first choice for the prevention of migraine. It should be reserved for patients with severe and disabling migraine, who have frequent attacks and who have not responded to pizotifen, propranolol and other drugs. Most of the potentially serious side effects can be avoided by observing the contraindications and by keeping the patient under careful and regular supervision. They should be in-structed to report any anginal pain, coldness, numbness or cramps in the limbs, or pains in the loins immediately. Appropriate laboratory investigations should be performed if signs of vascular insufficiency occur. Fibrotic reactions should not appear if treatment with methysergide is interrupted for four weeks every four to six months. As retroperitoneal fibrosis can develop without causing symp-toms, some physicians recommend urography every six to 12 months for patients taking methysergide over periods of years.

In the writer's experience methysergide has a better effect in the prevention of severe classic migraine than of the common form of the disease where emo-tional and other environmental triggers play a major aetiological role. It is not recommended for very anxious people with personality disorders — these people are also more likely to interpret various psychosomatic complaints as side effects of the drug. In recent years, the fear of side effects tended to be overemphasized. Severe migraineurs were denied the potentially great benefits of methysergide. It is hoped that the description of the good and undesirable effects of the drug will encourage physicians to prescribe it for selected patients with due caution.

3. Aspirin

It is now generally accepted that platelets aggregate more readily in the ma-jority of migrainous patients than in non-migrainous control subjects. They appear to be more aggregable during headache-free periods as well as before and during an attack. Platelets release serotonin when they aggregate. The drugs most effective for the prophylaxis of migraine, the antiserotonin-antihistaminic agents and methysergide, reduce spontaneous platelet aggregation. Propranolol was shown to have an antagonistic effect on serotonin, but its effect on platelet aggregation has not been reported.

Aspirin is a potent inhibitor of platelet aggregation as well as of prostaglandin synthesis. By preventing aggregation of platelets, aspirin inhibits serotonin release. Therefore, it may have an indirect antiserotonin effect. However, the writer decided not to include aspirin under the heading of antiserotonin agents, because of its other actions. It also inhibits secretion of serotonin by preventing synthesis of prostaglandin thromboxane A_2.

A double-blind trial of aspirin prophylaxis demonstrated that the drug achieved a better than 50% reduction in headache frequency in nine of 12 migraine patients (O'Neill and Mann, 1978). All three patients with classic migraine and six of the nine patients with common migraine responded. Three of five patients who obtained benefit from aspirin prophylaxis, and one of the two nonresponders tested, had hyperaggregable platelets. So far, no reports of large controlled studies of aspirin in the prevention of migraine headaches are available. The hypothesis that aggregation of platelets could add to the effect of constriction of small retinal and cerebral arterioles, and so produce the focal retinal and cerebral symptoms of migraine, is not unreasonable. It would be interesting to determine platelet aggregation in an adequate series of patients with classic migraine and in those patients who have attacks of migrainous angiospasm without ensuing headache. Further controlled clinical trials of the prophylactic effect of aspirin in these subgroups of migraineurs are needed.

The dose of aspirin in the clinical trial of O'Neill and Mann (1978) was 650mg twice daily. Aspirin is now frequently prescribed for the prevention of transient cerebral ischaemic attacks. It was recently suggested that smaller doses of soluble aspirin, of the order of 300mg once or twice daily, may suffice. Such smaller doses will reduce the incidence of gastric irritation which can also be controlled by antacids. Aspirin is generally a safe drug, but should not be prescribed for patients with a history of peptic ulcer or with any bleeding diathesis. A small number of people claim that they are intolerant to aspirin. Hypersensitivity in the form of skin rashes, acute angioneurotic oedema and bronchospasm occurs occasionally (Eadie and Tyrer, 1980).

Aspirin should not be given to patients taking anticoagulant drugs. Because of its antithrombotic and platelet inhibiting properties, it is advisable to withdraw regular aspirin medication before elective surgery or diagnostic procedures which involve arterial puncture.

4. Prostaglandin synthesis inhibitors

Although prostaglandin E_1 is a potent vasodilator and prostaglandins may have a role in modulating arterial tone, their plasma levels do not change during a migraine headache. Experimental work during the past ten years has shown that prostaglandins are not implicated in the pathogenesis of migraine. Clinical trials with drugs which inhibit prostaglandin synthesis, such as fenamates, indomethacin and naproxen, have established that they are no more effective than placebo for the prevention and treatment of migraine (Raskin, 1981).

The only exception is "chronic paroxysmal hemicrania" first described by Sjaastad and Dale (1974). This very rare headache entity has some similarities to the chronic form of cluster headache, but patients continue to experience from four to 12 short attacks of severe hemicrania every day without remission for years (see page 102). Treatment with indomethacin abolishes this pain immediately and completely, but it recurs if the drug is withdrawn. It is not certain if the dramatic response to indomethacin is due to inhibition of prostaglandin synthesis. As chronic paroxysmal hemicrania fails to respond to treatment with drugs which are effective in the management of other types of migraine and cluster headache, its pathogenesis appears to be quite different. Therefore, we have not included it among the migraine variants.

5. Amitriptyline

This tricyclic drug, widely used for the treatment of depressive states, was claimed to be effective for the prophylaxis of migraine in a few controlled clinical trials (Couch et al., 1976). The beneficial effect on migraine appears to be independent of the antidepressant action of the drug. It blocks the uptake of noradrenaline at catecholamine terminals and inhibits serotonin reuptake, but its mechanism of action in preventing migraine is not understood (Eadie and Tyrer, 1980). Amitriptyline has not gained wide acceptance for migraine prevention. A depressed mood is not unusual in people with frequent migrainous headaches and the drug should be prescribed mainly for patients with symptoms of depression, and after other drugs more effective in migraine prophylaxis have failed. The recommended dose ranges from 10mg to 75mg at night. As amitriptyline has a long half-life, its administration only at night is sufficient. The common side effects of sedation and anticholinergic actions (dry mouth, blurred vision, urine retention and constipation) may limit its acceptance by a proportion of patients. The drug should be taken for several weeks before its success or failure is assessed.

6. Monoamine oxidase (MAO) inhibitors

This group of drugs is used mainly for the treatment of psychotic depression refractory to other therapy. They irreversibly inhibit the enzyme monoamine oxidase (MAO) which inactivates various biogenic amines including serotonin (Eadie and Tyrer, 1980). The rationale for a trial of MAO inhibitors for migraine prophylaxis is that they would retard the breakdown of serotonin and would consequently maintain its peripheral action as a constrictor of cranial vessels. Anthony and Lance (1969) reported that the frequency of migraine headaches was reduced to less than 50% in 20 of 25 patients (80%) treated with phenelzine for periods of up to two years. It is not known if this high rate of good response was maintained in larger series of patients because physicians are generally reluctant to prescribe such a potentially dangerous drug for the management of migraine. If amine-containing foods are eaten by patients taking MAO inhibitors, severe hypertension may be induced by catecholamines and this has occasionally resulted in cerebral haemorrhage. The effects of MAO inhibitors persist for up to two weeks after the last dose because the MAO enzymes are irreversibly inhibited. Dangerous interactions with other drugs, including levodopa, centrally acting anticholinergics, tricyclic antidepressants, narcotics and alcohol, have been reported (Eadie and Tyrer, 1980). Therefore, phenelzine should be reserved for patients with severe migraine which has proved refractory to treatment with aspirin, propranolol, the antihistaminic-antiserotonin agents, and methysergide. Even then, it should be prescribed only for persons who can be trusted to adhere to the necessary diet restrictions and not take other drugs which may interact with phenelzine. They must be instructed not to consume amine-containing foods — these include: (i) certain cheeses; (ii) red wine; (iii) beer; (iv) broad bean pods; (v) meat extracts and vegetable extracts; (vi) chicken liver; (vii) yeast; (viii) yoghurt; and (ix) coffee. Close and regular supervision of the patient is essential. The dose of phenelzine used by Anthony and Lance (1969) is 15mg three times daily. Toxic effects include hypotension or hypertension, headache, convulsions, agitation, hallucinations, retention of urine and inhibition of ejaculation (Eadie and Tyrer, 1980)

We have dealt with all the drugs which from the results of controlled clinical trials may succeed in reducing the frequency and severity of migraine headaches. There are many other tablets, mixtures, herbs and potions which have been claimed, without controlled studies, to "cure" migraine. They do not require comment in a chapter which aims to describe a rationale for drug treatment.

The physician should first choose a drug with few side effects and ask the patient to take it for a minimum of eight weeks before deciding that it is not successful. If the patient has mild to moderate hypertension, propranolol would be the first choice; if a history of hay fever or other allergies is obtained, it would be wise to prescribe an antihistaminic-antiserotonin agent initially. Pizotifen seems to be the most effective drug in this group, but patients must be warned of weight gain if they cannot curtail their appetite. The value of daily aspirin is not clear yet, but it should be particularly considered for people with an angiospastic aura preceding the headache. Those who are depressed may benefit specifically from amitriptyline. Methysergide, though the best drug available for migraine prophylaxis, should be reserved for severe cases refractory to treatment with other drugs which have fewer potential side effects. Phenelzine is the last line of defence and should be used only if all else has failed.

The physician must then decide if drug treatment should be continuous or intermittent and tailored to the circumstances which have precipitated an individual person's attacks. For example, if migraine headaches occur predominantly during the premenstrual week, the selected drug may need to be taken only for seven to 10 days before and during menstruation. In women with premenstrual fluid retention, a diuretic taken at the appropriate time may contribute to an improvement in migraine. Ergotamine, combined with caffeine, with or without an antihistamine, may be taken before a stress situation (such as preparation for a dinner party or a shopping excursion) which has proved to be a trigger for a migraine attack.

Migraine Prophylaxis in Childhood

In Chapter 4 it was mentioned that about 4% of children between the ages of seven and 15 years suffer from genuine migraine. The attacks tend to occur more often, but are usually shorter in duration, than in adults. Parents bringing their child to the physician reasonably want to be reassured that no more serious or threatening cause of the recurring headaches has been overlooked. If the diagnosis can be established from the history and neurological examination, and from laboratory tests in selected cases, an attempt should be made to determine environmental factors which have contributed to the individual child's attacks. Some of these, such as specific foods or the excitement and exposure to flickering lights of a movie matinee, can be avoided, but the anxiety and stress of school examinations or the child's participation in sport and games on bright, sunny days, cannot be prevented. A child who experiences two or more migraine attacks per month should be given the benefit of preventive drug treatment. As antiserotonin agents may inhibit growth hormone release, they should be avoided or used with caution in children. The antihistaminic-antiserotonin agents (cyproheptadine, methdilazine) may also make the child drowsy and interfere with concentration at school.

Drugs with the least likelihood of side effects should be chosen. If the child has no history of asthma or frequent attacks of bronchitis, propranolol is the first choice. The dose of propranolol will vary with the age and size of the child; a dose of from 5mg to 20mg twice or three times daily is usually adequate. Treatment with propranolol should be maintained for at least eight weeks before there is any decision on its effectiveness. If successful prophylaxis is achieved, the dose can be gradually lowered until the minimum required is determined.

If propranolol fails or is not well tolerated, a small dose of a barbiturate, such as amylobarbitone 15mg twice daily, should be tried. The writer has found this treatment successful in a number of migrainous children. Side effects such as lethargy or irritability were never a problem. The mechanism of action of amylobarbitone for the prevention of childhood migraine is obscure, but Eadie and Tyrer (1980) state that anticonvulsant drugs, particularly phenytoin, succeed in preventing migrainous headaches in children up to the age of 12 years. The dose of phenytoin recommended is similar to that used in the treatment of epilepsy. It is of interest that anticonvulsant drugs are capable of preventing migraine in children, but not in adults. The relatively higher incidence of abnormal electroencephalographic tracings in migrainous children compared to adults does not provide a satisfactory explanation for this phenomenon. Administration of a compound preparation of phenobarbitone 20mg, ergotamine tartrate 0.3mg and belladonna alkaloids 0.1mg (Bellergal) often succeeds in reducing the frequency of migrainous headaches in children (Lance, 1972b). A dose of one tablet at night is usually sufficient. The writer had similar favourable experiences with Bellergal, and wonders if the phenobarbitone, a drug still widely used as an anticonvulsant, contained in the tablet may not be the essential active ingredient.

Drugs with potentially serious side effects, however rare, such as methysergide and phenelzine, should not be given to children. No information is so far available on the value of aspirin prophylaxis in children, but soluble aspirin in a 300mg to 600mg dose, combined with an antiemetic, such as 5mg to 10mg metoclopramide or 2.5mg to 5mg prochlorperazine maleate, is the treatment of choice for a migraine attack in children. Ergotamines, administered either by mouth or rectally, are very rarely needed during childhood and should be reserved for the uncommon, severe cases where aspirin and other simple analgesics have failed.

Non-Pharmacological Methods of Migraine Prophlaxis

We have shown earlier in this book that a great variety of events and stimuli in the external environment, as well as changes in the internal physiological milieu, are capable of bringing on an attack of common migraine. The results of experimental and clinical observations during the past 20 years permit the working hypothesis that migrainous persons differ from their more fortunate, non-migrainous fellows at all times, even during headache-free periods. The migraineur may have platelets which aggregate excessively, as well as permanent anomalies in both central and peripheral serotonergic function. Other vasoactive amines, as yet unknown, may also be involved. Many people who suffer from common migraine have a functional instability of the autonomic nervous system which may declare itself from childhood onwards and can affect the gastrointestinal and urogenital systems as well as the peripheral and cranial vessels. A person with such a permanent propensity to vasomotor dysregulation is constantly vulnerable and will develop a migrainous headache if certain triggers, which may be specific for an individual, ignite the quietly smouldering, but asymptomatic, cinders. Therefore, it is the duty of the attending physician to try and elucidate any environmental circumstances which may have contributed to the "explosion" of a migraine attack. This demands both patience and skill.

Some people state that their headaches are worse on hot and humid days, but little can be done to protect them from exposure to unfavourable climatic conditions. Many more find that glare, particularly bright light reflected from water, sand and snow will provoke an attack. A sunny day on the beach usually ends in a migraine headache. This can be prevented by wearing sunglasses, but the glaring headlights of oncoming cars when driving at night are more difficult to avoid. The flickering lights of a movie screen are a potent trigger. Migraineurs should avoid sitting in the front rows of the theatre. The distress of an attack should convince children that movie matinees are bad for them.

Since the lay press, particularly the periodicals widely read by women, has drawn attention to dietary items which can precipitate a migraine attack, many people have avoided chocolate, cheese, red wine and fried foods long before they consult their physician. While it is true that such foods can bring on an attack in individual people, it certainly does not apply to all migraineurs. Consumption of red wine, tyramine-containing foods, or a whole block of chocolate will often contribute to a vascular headache within a few hours or on the following morning. However, it is naive to prohibit such food for all migraine sufferers. Patients should be asked to record all foods and drinks consumed on the day before each migraine attack. In this manner, specific dietary items which may have contributed to that individual's attacks can be discovered. Through this approach one of the writer's patients found that apples were the cause of migraine. He remained entirely free of vascular headaches for years once he avoided apples. He then tested his observation, ate an apple and had a severe attack of migraine. Although apples are not one of the common foods which can provoke a vascular headache, this patient's experience demonstrates that the response of any individual can be highly specific. Red wine has acquired a bad reputation as migrainogenic, but many people report that even small quantities of any form of alcohol can result in an attack on the following morning.

Radioallergosorbent (RAST) tests may help to discover which foods provoke migraine in an individual person and they are less time consuming than elimination diets. In a group of 33 severe migraineurs, Monro *et al.* (1980) identified headache-provoking foods in 23 patients. Many of them were allergic to more than one group of foods. In all these patients, elimination of the offending food in the diet resulted in marked and rapid relief from migraine.

Oral contraceptives, and oestrogens taken after the menopause, may certainly aggravate migraine, but their importance has been overemphasized in the lay press, and possibly in the minds of many physicians. The only way to determine whether hormonal contraceptives have any influence on a particular woman's headaches is to withdraw them for at least three months and to compare the frequency and severity of her attacks during that time with their incidence while she was taking the hormone preparation. It is tragic, and also ridiculous, that some women are still subjected to hysterectomy in the hope that the resultant abolition of menstrual flow may improve migraine occurring mainly around the time of menstruation. Drugs for the prevention of migraine taken during the premenstrual week are more effective and less traumatic than pelvic surgery. The results of treatment with hormone preparations are usually disappointing.

A proportion of migraineurs recognize that their attacks will occur if they sleep in at weekends. Others have a vascular headache upon waking from a deep sleep. The mechanisms which contribute to this relationship between sleep and vascular headache are not understood. Most patients report headaches only if they rise late in the morning. However, headaches do not occur after an equal duration of sleep if they retired early and woke at the usual hour. This sequence of events is quickly recognized and is one of the migraine triggers most easily avoided.

This leaves us with stress, the most frequent and most important precipitant for common migraine. It is not intended to convey the impression that migraine is an essentially psychosomatic disorder, but patients' constitutions and personalities decide that they react to problems in their environment with changes in the cranial vessels, whereas non-migrainous persons may react to similar stress with alterations in blood pressure or disorders of gastrointestinal motility. An unstable autonomic nervous system, excessive aggregability of platelets or disorders of central or peripheral serotonergic mechanisms may be inherited along with the individual's personality structure.

Stress at work or at home, and concern over economic, social or political changes, are unavoidable. However, we have some means of modifying the magnitude of a person's reaction to stress and may thereby contribute to an improvement in vascular headaches. The aetiological role of stress is obviously important in common migraine. It has little significance for classic migraine and its variants.

Sedatives and tranquillizing drugs can help to tide a patient over an acutely stressful situation. However, they are better avoided for the prolonged treatment of chronic migraine. There is an increasing number of people who refuse to take tranquillizers, either fearing dependence or addiction, or interpreting the need for such drugs as an admission of a personality defect. People who find it difficult to relax, who admit to worrying excessively over trivial matters and who have recognized that many of their paroxysmal headaches are related to stressful situations can often be helped by hypnotherapy, relaxation exercises and biofeedback.

1. Behaviour therapy: Hypnosis, relaxation training and biofeedback

Earlier it was mentioned that many patients with common migraine also suffer from other clinical manifestations of an impaired regulation of the autonomic nervous system (page 14). These include: (i) cold hands and feet; (ii) dizziness and syncope; (iii) excessive changes in pulse rate and blood pressure in response to stress; (iv) nervous dyspepsia; and (v) dysmenorrhoea. Migraine may be regarded as a neurogenic vasomotor disorder with episodic changes in vascular calibre both in the internal and external carotid beds. Dalessio (1981) suggests that an incapacity to alter autonomic functions is a fundamental characteristic of migraine patients; they cannot alter their vasomotor responses in the same manner as non-migrainous people can.

Kudrow and Sutkus (1979) found from Minnesota Multiphasic Personality Inventory (MMPI) scores that patients with vascular headaches of migraine type tended to be less neurotic than those with muscle contraction and combined tension-vascular headaches. However, Dalessio (1981) suggests that this difference may be due to the frequent and longer pain-free intervals in migraine patients. In his series of 58 female migraineurs, the MMPI always showed a neurotic triad and indicated the patients' preoccupation with disease and their feelings of despair about its alleviation.

During the last 10 years, a number of reports have dealt with the success of various techniques of behaviour therapy for the relief of headache. Some of them describe a very small number of cases; most do not make a clear distinction between migraine and tension headache. These techniques do not lend themselves to controlled studies, such as single or double-blind trials. Many authors admit that good results may be partly attributed to the enthusiasm of the physician or psychologist and to the patients' anticipation of gaining relief at last from a new method of treatment which had not been tried before. Behaviour therapy requires more effort and co-operation from patients than the ingestion of drugs. In some cases, psychological resistance to this form of treatment is hard to overcome.

Hypnosis may be used as the first step. Subjects who can be hypnotized easily and who have a high hypnotic induction profile seem to fare better than those with a low profile. The patient is then taught procedures for inducing self-hypnosis. These involve relaxation, visual imagery, verbal reinforcement and direct suggestion. It may require from six to 12 sessions, each of 45 to 60 minutes duration, to make the patient competent in these techniques. They should then practise for at least 10 minutes two or three times each day. Tapes may facilitate the performance of relaxation exercises in the patient's home. Some psychologists claim that a combination of relaxation, desensitization and assertive therapy is more effective than relaxation alone. Desensitization consists of training in: (i) deep muscle relaxation; (ii) construction of anxiety hierarchies; and (iii) graduated pairing of imagined stimuli eliciting anxiety with the relaxed state. The patient is instructed to rehearse procedures designed to cope more effectively with personal problems.

Most people can be taught to exert voluntary control over some autonomic functions, such as raising the temperature of the skin of their finger or hands, by appropriate suggestions while they are in a self-hypnotized state. An appropriate suggestion might be the vivid imagination that they are warming their hands over a roaring fire or in a basin of warm water. Other autonomic functions, such as pulse rate and blood pressure, can also be modified during autohypnosis.

If a thermometer is strapped to the patient's finger and attached to a visible temperature recording gauge, the patient can observe the success of the auto-hypnotic efforts. More elaborate temperature feedback meters, programmed into a computer which produces a sound signal whenever the temperature is rising, can be used. These procedures are called biofeedback. It has been shown that a combination of autogenic training with biofeedback will enable a person to achieve voluntary control over some autonomic functions.

Other techniques record an electromyogram (EMG) from the patients' fore-heads, so that they can witness the relaxation of the frontalis muscle resulting from their deliberate efforts to relax. Another procedure, less frequently used in the treatment of headaches, requires a modified and simplified electroencephal-ographic machine with a brain wave analyser programmed into a computer. This produces a sound when the cerebral alpha rhythm is enhanced and becomes more prominent and regular.

Biofeedback systems, derived from either autonomic functions, EMG or electroencephalography, simply measure a particular physiological function and feed the information back to the individual as visual or auditory signals. Changes in the desired direction can be recognized and reinforced by the subject who must achieve some degree of voluntary control over the particular physiological function. While EMG biofeedback training has been mainly used in the treat-ment of muscle contraction (tension) headache, relief from vascular headaches of migraine type has been reported from biofeedback techniques designed to raise the skin temperatures of fingers, combined with autohypnosis and relaxation exercises.

The results of a trial of autogenic feedback training in a group of 75 headache patients, of whom 57 suffered from migraine, were reported by Sargent, Walters and Green (1973). Each patient was instructed in the use of a "temperature trainer" which showed the temperature of the mid-forehead and of the right index finger. Specific sets of phrases were used to foster relaxation of the whole body and to achieve warmth in the hands. Changes of temperature occurred more readily in the hands than in the forehead. The patients practised twice daily and recorded their success in relaxation and in warming the hand. The "temperature trainer" was withdrawn after the technique was mastered and patients subsequently used hand warming in an attempt to control attacks of migraine. Over a follow-up period ranging from one to three years, some 81% of the whole group of 75 headache patients showed significant improvement within 150 days of starting training in the autogenic feedback techniques. The degree of improvement varied.

Another study deals with 33 subjects suffering from migraine, randomly divided into three groups of 11 patients each. One group was treated by hypnosis and autohypnosis alone; the second was treated by biofeedback to raise hand temperature; and the third group was trained in biofeedback to enhance the cere-bral alpha rhythm. All three groups showed significant improvement in fre-quency and severity of migraine attacks. Across the three groups it was found that easily hypnotizable subjects fared better than those who had a low hypnotic induction profile (Andreychuk and Skriver, 1975). This may imply that the more suggestible subjects with high expectations of being helped are more likely to respond favourably to hypnosis and biofeedback treatment methods. This differential response of easily hypnotizable subjects has been referred to as the placebo response.

Anderson, Basker and Dalton (1975) compared the results of hypnotherapy (hypnosis and autohypnosis) in 23 migraine patients with 24 migraineurs who received 20mg prochlorperazine daily for prophylaxis. The trial was well designed and continued for one year. Although prochlorperazine reduces nausea, it was never shown by controlled trials to have any effect in the prevention or treatment of vascular headaches of migraine type. Therefore this trial really compares hypnotherapy with patients who received no potentially effective drug treatment. Hypnosis and autohypnosis reduced the frequency of attacks by over 75% and their severity by more than 50%; 10 of the 23 patients enjoyed a complete remission during the last three months of hypnotherapy. No significant improvement was reported by the patients treated with prochlorperazine.

A recent trial published by Friedman and Taub (1982) is concerned with 23 female migraine patients treated by a combination of hypnosis, autohypnosis and finger-warming by biofeedback procedures. Headache frequency, duration, intensity and requirements for pain-relieving drugs improved significantly in all 18 subjects who completed the six months follow-up period. It was found that the degree of improvement was independent of the patient's susceptibility to hypnosis and also independent of her ability to raise finger temperature. These authors conclude that screening for hypnotic susceptibility and elaborate training to achieve elevation of hand temperature may be unnecessary encumbrances and that a simple, non-instrumented technique of hypnosis and autohypnosis may suffice for the prevention of migraine headaches.

However, the findings of Dalessio (1981) do not agree entirely with the conclusions reached by Friedman and Taub (1982). Dalessio's study deals with 58 female migraine patients, 29 of them treated with propranolol and occasional analgesics, and the other 29 treated with a technique of progressive muscular relaxation combined with biofeedback training designed to raise the temperature of the middle finger on the headache side volitionally by at least 1°C within 15 minutes. The training period lasted approximately six weeks, but the time when the clinical results were evaluated is not stated. The incidence, intensity of headache and intake of pain relieving medication were recorded and patients who achieved at least a 50% reduction in two or all three of these parameters were rated as improved. In the biofeedback group, 16 subjects improved and 13 failed to respond; only 20 patients were available for evaluation in the propranolol plus analgesic group and nine of these improved. The neurotic triad configuration in the Minnesota Multiphasic Personality Inventory (MMPI) remained unaltered in all patients on medication (whether their condition was improved or unimproved) and in those patients who failed to improve on relaxation and biofeedback finger-warming techniques. A statistically significant change was seen in certain scales of the MMPI profile of the biofeedback improved subjects. This suggests that the psychoneurotic characteristics in migraineurs are an inherent feature of the aetiology of their migraine and cannot be attributed just to the pain experience. In the patients who responded to relaxation training and biofeedback, the psychoneurotic background improved concurrently with clinical improvement.

Dalessio (1981) suggests that the conditioned reflex characterized by dilation of the peripheral blood vessels of the hand and arm, and learned through biofeedback training, is a central requirement for migraine relief. As it is usually associated with slowing of the pulse rate, a general decrease of sympathetic tonic outflow occurs, not just the single conditioned autonomic response of digital vasodilation. This learned dilation of peripheral blood vessels in the hand and arm is apparently associated with a reduced blood flow in the supraorbital and superficial temporal arteries and is regarded as an adaptation-relaxation reflex. The use of this reflex will not only reduce the incidence and severity of migraine attacks; it can also abort an imminent headache.

On the basis of these observations, Dalessio (1981) proposes that psycho-neuroticism and a concomitant defect of central autonomic regulation may be an integral part of the migraine picture. Retraining of the autonomic nervous system, with the aim of decreasing sympathetic activity and teaching the patient to modify and correct at will the disturbed autonomic regulatory pattern in re-sponse to stress, can achieve improvement in migraine.

Some of the publications on the results of behaviour therapy provide criteria for the diagnosis of migraine, but none distinguish between classic and common migraine. Most have dealt with only a small number of patients. Follow-up ob-servations have been for only short periods after hypnotherapy or biofeedback techniques were completed. Controlled studies, similar to those applied to drug trials, cannot be undertaken. It is generally admitted that the placebo effects of hopeful anticipation and of the patients' suggestibility are difficult to assess. A brief summary of the techniques used and of the results of some trials has been given so that readers can make their own judgment.

Inevitably, hypnotherapy and biofeedback are sometimes practised by peo-ple who are not fully qualified and who may be over-enthusiastic in the inter-pretation of their results.

If we accept the concept of autonomic dysregulation as an aetiological back-ground for common migraine, then hypnotherapy and biofeedback with hand-warming procedures, initiated and taught by a well qualified therapist, will have a great deal to offer to a number of carefully selected patients. The guidelines for such selection include the following.

Guidelines for selection of patients for biofeedback or hypnotherapy

1. Patients with common migraine or with a combination of vascular and tension headaches.

2. Tense people where stress often precipitates attacks.

3. Concurrent symptoms of autonomic instability, such as vasomotor diz-ziness and faintness, attacks of palpitations, or wide fluctuations of blood pres-sure in response to stress.

4. The patient must be willing to participate in a prolonged treatment pro-gramme and to spend some time each day on autohypnosis and biofeedback exercises.

5. The patient must be informed and should accept that relief from headache may not occur for up to six months after the techniques have been mastered and practised properly.

Larger and better controlled trials are still needed, as well as more well-trained hypnotherapists. Time and cost can be reduced by teaching relaxation in classes or groups. The equipment used for feedback temperature training need not be complex nor expensive.

With the widespread, but often exaggerated and unjustified, fear of drugs and their side effects, and as a result of the apparent difficulty some doctors experience in communicating with patients, the concept of "alternative" medicine has gained wide publicity and some acceptance. Cervical manipulation and acupuncture may be included in the large umbrella of "alternative" treatments because neither lends itself to a rational scientific explanation for the prevention of migraine.

2. Cervical manipulation

Muscle contraction (tension) headaches and the combined form of "tension-vascular" headache frequently respond to cervical manipulation whether this is performed by an interested and enthusiastic medical practitioner or by a chiropractor. At many meetings or seminars dealing with migraine, some member of the audience will rise during discussion time and assert that he or she has "cured" thousands of migraineurs completely and permanently by cervical manipulation. These statements do not provide diagnostic criteria, duration of follow-up periods, or any of the data demanded by orthodox medicine for the evaluation of controlled clinical trials.

In a critical review of headaches and cervical manipulation, Bogduk (1979) points out that upper cervical lesions can cause headaches. The anatomical substrate is the innervation of the joints and ligaments of the upper three cervical vertebrae by branches of the first, second and third cervical spinal roots. As these converge centrally with the spinal nucleus of the trigeminal nerve, pain can be referred to the orbit and forehead. Reduced mobility of the upper cervical spine and minor subluxations in cervical zygapophyseal joints may thus cause frontal and periorbital headache amenable to manipulative therapy. This may occur in rheumatoid arthritis, but the headache has none of the periodicity and clinical characteristics of common migraine or any other variety of the migraine syndrome. The assumption that the vertebral artery or its sympathetic plexus can be "irritated" by osteophytes from the uncovertebral region or lateral disc protrusions has never been substantiated. It is naive to propose that the extremely rare condition of "basilar" migraine, where attacks occur no more than once or twice a year, could be caused by a chronic and persistent compression or irritation of the vertebral artery by degenerated joints or discs in the cervical spine. It must be emphasized again that pain in the head can be referred only from the upper three cervical sensory roots. Therefore, it is amazing that many middle-aged patients come to the neurologist for the treatment of vascular headaches of migraine type bearing X-ray films of the cervical spine which had been ordered for the diagnostic investigation of their migraine. Many of these X-ray films will show narrowing of disc spaces in the mid-cervical region, as is so common during and after middle age. Most of these patients had been subjected to cervical manipulation by medical practitioners, physiotherapists or chiropractors, but the placebo effect of hopeful anticipation of relief had worn off and so, disillusioned but wiser, they came to seek help from a more rational and scientific therapeutic approach.

A well designed, controlled study of the effect of cervical manipulation in the treatment of migraine was reported by Parker, Tupling and Pryor (1978). Eighty-five volunteers with a diagnosis of migraine made by neurologists from generally accepted criteria were randomly allocated to three treatment groups. One group was treated with cervical manipulation performed by a medical practitioner or physiotherapist. Patients in the second group received cervical manipulation from a chiropractor (manipulation is defined as a sudden thrust to a cervical joint, which is thus forced beyond its normal range of movement). The third group of patients, the control group, was treated by cervical "mobilization" where the therapists induce only small oscillatory movements to the cervical joints within their normal range. The trial extended over six months. In the first pretreatment phase of two months, the frequency, duration, severity and degree of disability caused by each migraine attack were recorded. During the second phase patients received either cervical manipulation or mobilization on a twice-weekly average for two months. Drug therapy for migraine, which the patients had used before the trial, was not altered during the study. The third or post-treatment phase of the trial also extended over two months. The frequency, duration, severity and disability caused by migraine attacks were again recorded. The age of patients, the duration and severity of migraine, and the patients' neuroticism scores calculated from the Eysenck Personality Inventory were similar in the three groups. X-ray examinations of the cervical spine revealed degenerative changes in 42% of patients. A further 13% showed radiological criteria of movement restriction. These were also equally represented in the three treatment groups. For the whole sample, migraine symptoms were reduced, including a 28% reduction in the frequency of attacks. This proportion of improvement is similar to that reported from placebo drugs used as controls in therapeutic trials. No difference in outcome was found between those patients who received cervical manipulation performed by an orthodox therapist or a chiropractor, and those who were in the control group which received cervical mobilization. Patients treated by chiropractors reported a greater reduction in pain intensity, but not in frequency, duration or degree of disability induced by the migraine attacks. The authors comment that the greater enthusiasm of the chiropractors may have accounted for the better improvement in pain intensity of their patients, a placebo effect to which we have already referred in the discussion of behaviour therapy. It is also of interest that patients with degenerative changes in X-ray examinations of the cervical spine did not respond better to manipulation or mobilization than those without such radiological abnormalities.

The distress of a severe and protracted vascular headache of migraine type may cause secondary excessive contraction of the posterior cervical muscles. A suboccipital pain will then appear in addition to the migrainous headache. This pain may outlast the migraine attack and can sometimes be alleviated by cervical mobilization or manipulation, or by administration of muscle relaxing drugs such as diazepam. Apart from this (in the writer's opinion) cervical manipulation has no place in the treatment of migraine.

3. Acupuncture

Although acupuncture is now widely practised and has aroused great expectations among the disciples of "alternative" medicine, no acupuncture points or regions specific for the treatment of migraine have been proposed and no controlled trials of the success of acupuncture for the prevention and treatment of migraine are available. However, there is no dearth of unsubstantiated and unscientific hypotheses which claim that acupuncture triggers off a series of local events altering the permeability of cell membranes by liberating serotonin, bradykinin, histamine and prostaglandins. It is further claimed that stimulation of the major acupuncture points will release specific corticosteroids and produce vasoconstriction (Kim, 1975). None of these hypotheses has been supported by experimental evidence and none can be reconciled with current knowledge of the pathogenesis of migraine. It is conceivable that any beneficial effect of acupuncture, if such occurs, may be mediated by the brain's neuropeptides and opiate receptors, such as encephalins and endorphins, which are stimulated by the insertion and movement of the acupuncture needles.

As with behaviour therapy and cervical manipulation, the patient's anticipation of success, enhanced by the optimistic and forceful promises of the acupuncturist, may have an initial placebo effect. However, this rarely persists for longer than a few weeks after the course of treatment is completed. This writer has not yet seen a person who enjoyed a lasting reduction in the frequency, duration or severity of migraine headaches from acupuncture treatment. However, patients who are anxious to try acupuncture should be encouraged to proceed, lest they are left with a doubt that an avenue of relief, which had been of benefit to some of their friends with other painful conditions, had not been explored.

The data presented on the various treatment modalities available for the prevention of migraine permit the following conclusions.

Conclusions about various treatment modalities

1. Drug treatment offers the best chance of success. Specific drugs have to be selected for each patient depending on the type and severity of migraine. The most suitable drug can often be determined only by trial and error.

2. Environmental factors recognized as contributing to the occurrence of a migraine attack should be avoided as far as possible.

3. Patients with common migraine where stress is a major trigger, and those who are reluctant to take pharmaceutical preparations, should be referred to behaviour therapists.

4. The wish of a person to try cervical manipulation or acupuncture should be respected; if these procedures fail, the patient may be more willing to accept prophylaxis with pharmacological agents.

In the initial discussion about preventive measures with each patient, it must be pointed out that complete cure should not be anticipated and that only a reduction in the frequency and severity of migraine can be hoped for. Occasional attacks will continue to occur.

Treatment of the Acute Migraine Attack

The treatment of a migraine attack aims at reducing pain and preventing or diminishing nausea and vomiting. As the dilating extracranial arteries rapidly become more rigid and resistant to vasoconstrictor agents, and as gastric atony develops quickly and interferes with the absorption of ingested drugs from the small intestine, it is essential for the patient to *take medications at the very onset of an attack.* This is most easily achieved in classic migraine when patients should be instructed to take tablets during the aura. The ensuing headache can often be prevented or greatly reduced in intensity. The importance of early treatment must be stressed in the initial discussion with each patient as many people are reluctant to take medication before the pain has become severe. At that stage of a migraine attack, oral drugs are absorbed poorly and the patient may be forced to take large doses of strong analgesics without much benefit. If a migraine headache is present on waking, drugs taken by mouth are unlikely to produce significant relief.

Aspirin

Aspirin is recommended as the first line of treatment. As speed of action is essential, one of the soluble aspirins should be prescribed. The patient should be instructed to dissolve it in a small volume of water before swallowing it. A relatively large dose of 600mg to 900mg or more of soluble aspirin should be taken because gastric absorption is probably delayed and incomplete. Metoclopramide hydrochloride in a 10mg dose should be taken together with soluble aspirin. This will increase gastric motility and help the passage of aspirin into the small intestine where it can be absorbed. Metoclopramide also relieves nausea and vomiting but, like aspirin, is not absorbed well once gastric atony has developed in the later stages of a migraine attack.

If the headache continues, the patient may take compound preparations of aspirin with codeine or dextropropoxyphene at intervals of four hours, but the poor absorption of all orally ingested drugs will interfere with their efficacy.

Aspirin acts not only as an analgesic but also prevents aggregation of platelets, thereby inhibiting release of serotonin. It is also a potent inhibitor of prostaglandin synthesis. Therefore, aspirin may act on several components which contribute to the genesis of a migraine attack and curtail its progression.

There are no known drugs for the treatment of the angiospastic aura which precedes headache. A rapidly acting vasodilator, such as sublingual glyceryl trinitrate, may shorten the visual or focal cerebral symptoms, but usually increases the intensity of the ensuing headache.

If aspirin has failed to provide relief, or if it is not tolerated, ergotamines are the next line of treatment.

Ergotamine

Ergotamine has been used for almost 60 years to treat migraine. It is an alkaloid derived from a fungus which grows on rye and other grain crops and it is generally prescribed as the tartrate salt. It is a partial alpha-adrenergic agonist and a potent vasoconstrictor agent with a selective action in the carotid bed. Regional cerebral blood flow studies in humans have shown that therapeutic doses of ergotamine constrict the external, but not the internal, carotid system (references cited by Eadie and Tyrer, 1980). While ergotamine acts as a vasoconstrictor when vessels are dilated and vascular resistance is low, it may produce vasodilation when vascular resistance is increased. This explains why both the early angiospastic and the later vasodilator phases of a migraine attack may respond to the drug (Raskin, 1981). The drug also inhibits the reuptake of norepinephrine and reduces the increased rate of platelet aggregation induced by serotonin (American Hospital Formulary Service, 1981).

Few data are available on the pharmacokinetics, absorption and elimination of ergotamine because of the difficulty in obtaining sufficiently sensitive assays. The discrepancy between the effective oral dose of 2mg to 4mg and intravenous dose of 0.25mg to 0.5mg in the treatment of migraine suggests that the drug is poorly absorbed from the alimentary tract or that there is a substantial first-pass metabolism in the gut wall and liver (Eadie and Tyrer, 1980). Ergotamine absorption from the alimentary tract may be enhanced by the simultaneous presence of caffeine (Fanchamps, 1976). Aellig and Nuesch (1977) found that the maximum plasma concentration of tritium-labelled ergotamine was reached two hours after an oral dose and that elimination half-lives were 1.9 ± 0.6 hours (alpha-phase) and 21 ± 4 hours (beta-phase). Intramuscular administration achieved the highest and longest lasting plasma ergotamine concentration. Plasma levels were a little higher after rectal administration than after oral administration (Ala-Hurula *et al.*, 1979). Sutherland *et al.* (1974) reported that buccal absorption of ergotamine was unlikely to yield therapeutic plasma levels. The degree of absorption from inhaled ergotamine has not been adequately studied, but clinical observations have indicated that the inhalant mode of administration is not very successful in the treatment of migraine.

The common side effects of ergotamine include nausea, vomiting and spasm of the peripheral arteries. These effects are dose-related, though nausea may occur even after small doses. The emetic action is attributed to stimulation of chemoreceptor zones in the medulla. Ergotamine may also cause cramps in the abdomen and legs, coronary artery spasm and venous thrombosis. Gangrene of the extremities has been reported after prolonged use. Very rarely, gangrene may occur in patients on low doses, suggesting an idiosyncratic mechanism. Although ergotamine has an oxytocic effect, it has not been used to induce abortion and there is no clear evidence that it is dysmorphogenic in humans (Eadie and Tyrer, 1980).

Ergotamine must be used with caution in patients with coronary or peripheral arterial disease and in those with a history of venous thrombosis. The relatively small doses required for an attack of migraine are unlikely to cause uterine contractions, so its use during pregnancy is not necessarily contraindicated. Severe cramps in the lower limbs very rarely occur in individuals who are abnormally sensitive to the vasospastic effects of the drug; ergotamines should not be prescribed again for such people.

Ergotamine is available as sublingual tablets containing either 1mg or 2mg of the active drug, or in compound preparations which contain 1mg ergotamine tartrate with 100mg caffeine (Cafergot and several other brands offered by the pharmaceutical industry in various countries). Antihistamines, such as cyclizine hydrochloride or diphenhydramine hydrochloride have been added to some preparations containing 1mg or 2mg ergotamine tartrate and 100mg caffeine, presumably on the assumption that the antihistamine would control nausea and vomiting caused by either the migraine attack itself or the administered ergotamine. In clinical practice this assumption has not been substantiated, but the antihistamine content of the tablets may make the patient more tired and drowsy.

Selby and Lance (1960) found that 47% of 263 migraine patients obtained rapid and marked relief from headache after oral, sublingual or parenteral administration of ergotamine. In a further 34% of these patients, only a proportion of attacks were aborted or headache of diminished severity continued. Other reports published before 1960 have quoted comparable results.

Unless any of the contraindications mentioned above exist, tablets containing ergotamine tartrate and caffeine should be prescribed if aspirin failed to relieve headache in previous attacks. The initial dose should be 1mg to 2mg ergotamine; this can be repeated after half to one hour. If small doses do not cause nausea, the patient should take 3mg to 4mg ergotamine as the initial dose. It must be explained to the patient that the drug will prevent or reduce headache only if taken at the very beginning of an attack, and preferably during the aura. It is only at that stage that ergotamine can be absorbed from the gut and that the distended extracranial vessels will respond to its vasoconstrictive action. Metoclopramide in a dose of 10mg should be taken together with the compound tablet of ergotamine and caffeine. Metoclopramide will assist with the absorption of ergotamine as well as preventing nausea. Other antiemetic drugs can be used if metoclopramide is not well tolerated. Prochlorperazine (5mg), thiethylperazine (6.5mg) or meclozine (25mg) can be tried and will often prevent vomiting. However, unlike metoclopramide, these agents do not improve gastric motility or facilitate the absorption of ergotamine.

If the patient wakes with a migrainous headache, if nausea occurs very early in the attack, or if the tablets cannot be taken until the headache is well advanced, ergotamine should be administered by the rectal route rather than oral route. Cafergot-PB suppositories (available in Australia) contain 2mg ergotamine tartrate, 100mg caffeine, 0.25mg alkaloids of belladonna and 100mg itobarbitone. There is little need for belladonna or the barbiturate except for patients who want to sleep. In the USA, Cafergot suppositories contain only 2mg ergotamine and 100mg caffeine which appears to be a more satisfactory formulation for most people. Though there is some variation between individuals, mean plasma ergotamine levels are higher after rectal administration than after oral administration of the drug. Suppositories, like tablets, must be used as early as possible in an attack and, if necessary, a second suppository may be inserted one or two hours after the first. If nausea and vomiting are troublesome a 25mg prochlorperazine or 6.5mg thiethylperazine suppository should be used a few minutes after the ergotamine suppository. It is advisable to store suppositories at temperatures below 25°C.

Persons who are averse to using rectal suppositories may prefer to try sublingual tablets of ergotamine tartrate or oral inhalation from a metered spray, but there are no results of studies available to determine if adequate plasma levels of ergotamine are reached by these routes of administration. In the writer's experience, neither sublingual nor inhalant ergotamine has been very effective for the treatment of migraine.

Patients should try and determine the dose of ergotamine tablets or suppositories they need to relieve their headache during several attacks and then take the minimal effective dose at the very onset of subsequent attacks. The total oral or rectal dose should not exceed 6mg in 24 hours or 10mg in one week. As methysergide also has vasoconstrictor effects, doses of ergotamine tartrate should be decreased by about 50% and the frequency of its administration kept to a minimum if the patient takes methysergide regularly for migraine prophylaxis.

Parenteral administration of ergotamine results in the highest and longest lasting plasma levels (Ala-Hurula *et al.,* 1979). The injectable form of ergotamine tartrate was withdrawn from the market recently, but dihydroergotamine mesylate is available in 1ml ampoules containing 1mg of the drug. Dihydroergotamine is a semisynthetic ergot alkaloid, which has less vasoconstrictor action, but more alpha-adrenergic blocking activity, than ergotamine. Its actions are otherwise similar to those described for ergotamine. It has less oxytocic effect and may cause less nausea and vomiting than ergotamine. Peak plasma levels are attained 45 minutes after subcutaneous administration. If the drug is given by intramuscular or intravenous injection peak levels will be reached sooner.

The duration of action is three to four hours after intramuscular administration. Although severe vasospasm is less likely to occur from dihydroergotamine than from ergotamine, it should not be used in patients with peripheral vascular or coronary heart disease. Some people may complain of muscle pains in the limbs, precordial distress or numbness and paraesthesia in the fingers and toes after injections of dihydroergotamine (American Hospital Formulary Service, 1981).

The drug is more effective if administered as soon as possible after the onset of a vascular headache. The dose of dihydroergotamine is 1mg preferably by intramuscular injection. This dose can be repeated twice at hourly intervals. Once the patient has determined the total dose required from the experience of several attacks, a dose of 2mg to 3mg dihydroergotamine can be given at the onset of future vascular headaches. An injection of 10mg metoclopramide or a suppository of prochlorperazine or thiethylperazine will relieve nausea and vomiting. If injections of dihydroergotamine effectively control the vascular headache, while oral, inhalant or rectal ergotamines have failed, patients should be taught to administer the injections to themselves. If millions of diabetics throughout the world can learn to give themselves injections of insulin, there is no reason why migraineurs cannot be taught to inject dihydroergotamine. The subcutaneous route, though less effective than the intramuscular, is still preferable to tablets or suppositories. It is very rarely possible for the family physician to come within minutes and administer the injection at the early stage of a migraine attack when it will have its best effect.

Ergotamines in any form are unlikely to help if administered an hour or longer after the vascular headache began. Analgesics, such as combinations of aspirin or paracetamol with codeine, or dextropropoxyphene hydrochloride, are then needed. Some individuals who tolerate oral or rectal ergotamines find that the addition of these analgesics at the beginning of an attack provides the best relief. If at all possible, patients should lie down and rest in a cool, darkened room until the headache has abated. It must also be explained that a severe migraine attack and its treatment with ergotamines and analgesics will leave them listless and exhausted for several hours after the pain has disappeared.

Some migraineurs have occasional attacks when the headache fails to respond to the usual treatment and becomes so intense that it is described as intolerable. Then, the attending physician may have to administer narcotic analgesics such as pethidine, methadone or pentazocine. Morphine should be avoided because it is likely to cause or aggravate vomiting. Individuals who are emotionally unstable, or who have a poor tolerance to any pain, may demand such injections too often, but astute physicians who know their patients well will soon recognize those patients with a high risk of drug dependence or addiction. In a recurring disease, such as migraine, the risk of drug addiction must always be in the physician's mind.

A secondary muscle contraction headache resulting from the pain and stress of a vascular headache may develop and persist for several hours or days after the termination of the migraine attack. This can be treated with a combination of analgesics and diazepam.

Very rarely, true migraine can continue for several days or weeks instead of the usual 24 to 36 hours. This condition, called status migrainosus by some writers, is difficult to treat. There is a limit to the number of injections of narcotic analgesics which can be given, and it may be advisable to try and keep the patient asleep for long periods with large doses of benzodiazepines or barbiturates. In such cases it may be best to admit the patient to hospital for a complete rest from the inevitable stresses of the domestic environment. If ergotamines and analgesics fail, a course of treatment with corticosteroids, such as 10mg prednisone orally administered three or four times a day, or injections of 2mg to 4mg dexamethasone every eight hours, should be tried. Analgesics are continued in adequate doses until the steroids become effective. Once the migraine status has abated the dose of steroids can be reduced fairly rapidly. Their mode of action in this condition is unknown (Eadie and Tyrer, 1980).

At times, people who experience no side effects from ergot preparations and who remain constantly afraid of an impending migraine attack will take 2mg to 3mg ergotamine orally every day and become habituated to the drug. Their intake of ergotamines is consistently close to or in excess of the recommended maximum dose of 10mg to 12mg per week. As the effect of each dose wears off, a rebound headache occurs and more ergotamine is taken thus producing a vicious circle. These patients then complain of a constant, generalized headache, malaise and tiredness. The symptoms of ergotamine abuse can be treated only by withdrawal of the drug, which results in a more severe headache requiring treatment with strong analgesics and sedatives or admission to hospital for a few days. If the patient has taken a compound preparation of ergotamine and caffeine, the withdrawal of caffeine may contribute to the ensuing protracted pain in the head. Withdrawal symptoms and re-emergence of vascular headaches can be treated with propranolol, pizotifen or methysergide. If patients can be made to understand that excessive doses of ergotamine had caused their symptoms, they can later be allowed to use small doses of ergotamine again, but only at the onset of future migraine attacks.

Persons who suffer from both vascular and muscle contraction headache (tension-vascular headache) may also report that some pain in the head is virtually constant. Details of drug consumption will easily distinguish this condition from ergotamine abuse, but a painstaking history is necessary to decide how many of the headaches are migrainous and how many are due to muscle contraction. Both conditions must be treated. The tension headaches can be treated with psychotherapy, relaxation exercises, cervical mobilization, and administration of diazepam or other minor tranquillizers and the migrainous vascular headaches can be treated with the drugs described above for prophylaxis and for management of an acute attack.

The treatment of complicated migraine, whether basilar, hemiparaesthetic, hemiplegic or ophthalmoplegic, does not differ significantly from the therapy for common or classic migraine described above. Soluble aspirin, which reduces platelet aggregation, can be administered in an attempt to lessen the severity and duration of symptoms resulting from vasoconstriction in the retinal, carotid or basilar circulation, but, so far, no treatment is known to accelerate recovery from ophthalmoplegia. Eadie and Tyrer (1980) state that sustained treatment with orally administered anticonvulsants, particularly phenytoin, in doses similar to or lower than those used for epilepsy, is almost always effective in preventing these uncommon migraine variants. As experimental work has suggested that ergotamines dilate constricted intracranial vessels (Raskin, 1981), they can be used safely for the treatment of the headache phase of an attack of complicated migraine.

Prevention and Treatment of Cluster Headache

Theories of pathogenesis and clinical features of cluster headache were described in Chapter 4. In recent years two varieties of cluster headache have been distinguished.

1. Episodic, where paroxysms of severe unilateral headache occur once or several times each day during clusters lasting from two to 10 weeks and occasionally longer, but always separated by intervals of complete freedom from headache which can continue for months or years.

2. Chronic, where the clinical characteristics of headache are identical to the episodic type, but the attacks occur daily and haphazardly for months or years without headache-free intervals. The chronic form accounts for only 5% to 6% of all cluster headaches and may develop in patients who have suffered from the episodic variety for several years.

In contrast to common migraine there are no significant environmental factors which contribute to the occurrence of cluster headaches. A few patients seem to have clusters at the same time each year which would suggest exposure to a seasonal external allergen, but, in the majority of cases, no such predictable seasonal incidence can be established. In some people, changes in their sleep-wake pattern, excessive physical activity, excitement or anger were thought to have precipitated a cluster, but similar alterations in their lifestyles occurred at other times and they remained free of headache. Alcohol will trigger a headache paroxysm during a cluster, but not during a headache-free period. No other items of diet have been implicated. Hypnotherapy, relaxation training, biofeedback and cervical manipulation were found to have no effect in the management of cluster headache.

Several pharmaceutical preparations are available to prevent or at least reduce the intensity of the very severe paroxysmal pain during a cluster. In view of the prolonged pain-free intervals in the more common episodic variety of cluster headache, prophylactic treatment is started only as each cluster begins and is continued for several weeks until the cluster has come to its natural termination.

The drugs used for the prevention of episodic cluster headaches include ergotamines, methysergide, pizotifen, corticosteroids and lithium carbonate.

Ergotamines

It is generally accepted that extracranial vasodilation, mainly in the periorbital region, contributes to the pain of cluster headache. Sakai and Meyer (1979) have shown that there is also a marked increase in cerebral blood flow and that this is more pronounced on the side contralateral to the headache during a cluster attack. Ergotamine is the most effective extracranial vasoconstrictor agent. Its oral administration for the prevention of cluster headache was first reported by Ekbom in 1947. Symonds (1956a) was the first to observe the good effect of injections of 0.25mg to 0.5mg ergotamine tartrate two or three times daily; patients learned to administer these to themselves during a cluster. As some people resent the inconvenience of hypodermic or intramuscular injections, oral, sublingual or aerosol inhalant preparations of ergotamine were more widely used. These provided significant relief in 79% of the first 100 patients treated by Kudrow (1980). Oral ergotamine prophylaxis was not so successful in this writer's patients who took 1mg ergotamine tartrate morning and evening. In view of the extreme severity of pain, most sufferers were quite happy to inject themselves with 0.25mg to 0.5mg ergotamine tartrate subcutaneously or intramuscularly twice daily or at night if the attacks were purely nocturnal. At the end of each week, the injections were omitted for one day, so that the patient could discover if the cluster had ended. Parenterally administered ergotamine was prescribed only if oral or sublingual preparations had failed; this method afforded complete relief in all but two of about 30 patients with "episodic" cluster headache. The explanation for the better effect of parenteral administration compared with oral administration of ergotamine tartrate may be found in the higher and longer lasting plasma concentrations of the drug after intramuscular injection than after oral or rectal administration (Ala-Hurula et al., 1979). The results of plasma radioactivity studies suggest that the drug has a "fast" half-life of from five to six hours and a "slow" half-life of from 30 to 35 hours (Eadie and Tyrer, 1980). Injections of 0.5mg to 1mg dihydroergotamine mesylate in the morning and at night should now be used in place of ergotamine tartrate, which is no longer available. Dihydroergotamine is somewhat less liable than ergotamine tartrate to cause side effects of nausea, vomiting or pain and paraesthesia in the limbs due to peripheral vasoconstriction.

For the prophylaxis of cluster headache by the oral route, compound preparations containing 1mg to 2mg ergotamine tartrate and 100mg caffeine are recommended instead of ertogamine tartrate alone. As buccal absorption of ergotamine in humans appears to be an inefficient process (Sutherland et al., 1974), sublingual or inhalant preparations of the drug are less likely to prevent cluster headache than injections, tablets or rectal suppositories.

It is surprising how rarely symptoms of ergotism, such as pain, pallor and paraesthesia in the extremities, appear even after continuous use of ergotamine preparations for several weeks for prophylaxis of cluster headache. Withdrawal of the drug abolishes the symptoms rapidly in almost all cases, but it is essential to keep the patient under close and regular supervision. As mentioned earlier, ergotamine preparations should not be prescribed for patients with peripheral vascular or coronary artery disease, severe hypertension or hepatic or renal impairment. As cluster headaches predominate in males, their occurrence during pregnancy is very rare. In spite of the known oxytocic effects of ergotamines they may not be absolutely contraindicated in selected, pregnant patients. The potential side effects of all drugs which can contribute to prevention must then be weighed against the suffering of the mother.

Methysergide

This drug is effective for the prevention of the episodic type of cluster headache in from 65% to 77% of patients, but tends to lose its effect in subsequent clusters in about 20% of patients (Kudrow, 1980). Methysergide appears to be of no benefit to patients suffering from the chronic variety of cluster headache.

The dose of methysergide recommended for a bout of episodic cluster headache ranges from 6mg to 8mg daily. This is larger than the dose commonly employed for the prevention of migraine. As the drug is taken only during the two to ten weeks of a cluster, the risk of retroperitoneal, cardiac or pulmonary fibrosis is very low. However, other side effects of methysergide discussed earlier in this chapter may make it impossible for a patient to continue taking a dose adequate for prophylaxis.

Pizotifen

This antihistaminic, antiserotonin agent occasionally helps in preventing attacks during a cluster, but it is less effective than ergotamines, methysergide, corticosteroids and lithium carbonate. Therefore, it is not a drug of first choice. However, it should be tried in patients who cannot tolerate the other drugs. The pharmacology of pizotifen was described earlier. The recommended dose is 1mg of base (two tablets) two or three times daily. Common side effects include weight gain and drowsiness.

The mode of action of methysergide or pizotifen in the prevention of cluster headache is unknown. Plasma levels of serotonin do not fall during an attack of cluster headache. Methysergide may act by inhibiting histamine release by mast cells or by reducing the permeability of small blood vessels. The antihistaminic effect of pizotifen may be more important than its antiserotonin action, but other antihistamine drugs such as cyproheptadine or methdilazine were found to have no effect for prevention or treatment of cluster headache.

Corticosteroids

It is likely that the success of treatment with adrenal corticosteroids in immune complex diseases first motivated the trial of these agents for cluster headache prophylaxis. It was shown that whole blood levels of histamine rise significantly during an attack of cluster headache. It is known that corticosteroids inhibit histamine formation by reducing the activity of the enzyme histidine decarboxylase. However, blockade of histamine H_1 receptors with chlorpheniramine and of H_2 receptors with cimetidine does not influence the course of cluster headache. These drugs act only on circulating histamine and not on the amine formed and active at tissue level.

Jammes (1975) reported the first controlled study of prednisone for the prophylaxis of cluster headache. In a group of 77 patients with the episodic variety of the disease who had not responded to treatment with methysergide Kudrow (1980) reported marked relief from attacks in 76.6% and partial improvement in a further 11.7% of patients. The results of treatment with prednisone in the chronic type of cluster headache were not quite as spectacular, but still encouraging; of 15 patients, six obtained marked improvement and a further five improved partially.

Corticosteroids are now one of the first lines of treatment for prevention of episodic cluster headache, but their mode of action in this condition remains unknown. Dosage schedules vary with different physicians. Kudrow (1980) recommends a course of treatment extending over three weeks, beginning with 40mg prednisone daily for the first five days, 30mg for the next five days, 20mg for four days, 15mg for three days, 10mg for two days, and 5mg for the last two days.

Side effects include insomnia, mood changes and fluid retention, but these are relatively minor and resolve when the course of steroid treatment is completed. If the headache paroxysms are mainly nocturnal, an orally administered ergotamine preparation can be added and should be taken before going to bed.

Corticosteroids must be used with caution in patients who suffer from hypertension, infections, diabetes or peptic ulcer. Kudrow (1980) has seen two patients in whom diverticula of the colon perforated during steroid treatment.

If the paroxysms of cluster headache continue, a second course of prednisone in doses similar to the first can be prescribed after an interval of one week without steroids.

Lithium

Cluster headache is a cyclic disorder in which the attacks of headache may occur at the same time each day or night with clockwork regularity. As lithium had been found to be effective in the treatment of cyclic affective disorders, Ekbom (1974) decided to investigate the effect of lithium for the prevention of cluster headache. The results were encouraging, particularly in a small group of three patients with the chronic type of the disease. Kudrow (1977) then treated 32 patients with chronic cluster headache (either primary or following on a past history of the episodic type of the disease) for a period of 32 weeks. All these patients had been resistant to, or intolerant of, ergotamine, methysergide and prednisone. Of the 28 patients who completed this study, 14 achieved a greater than 90% improvement in headache frequency and intensity and a further 11 patients obtained improvement of from 60% to 90%. Some of the people whose condition improved with lithium therapy continued to experience bouts of mild cluster headache daily for three or four days every three to six weeks. A few had occasional severe attacks, even while remaining on the same maintenance dose. Lithium did not prevent attacks induced by alcohol.

The dose of lithium carbonate used by Kudrow, and by others who reported similar rates of success, ranged from 600mg to 900mg per day. Serum lithium levels should not be allowed to exceed 1.2mmol/L. It was found that lower maintenance doses often sufficed after the 12th week of treatment. The drug should not be given to patients taking diuretics or on a low salt diet.

Side effects from lithium therapy include fairly severe, throbbing occipital headache which can last for from six to 12 hours and recur, so that treatment cannot be continued. Other relatively minor side effects, such as tremor, decreased concentration and memory, insomnia, lethargy, lightheadedness, diarrhoea, abdominal pain and vomiting, need not interfere with continuing lithium therapy. Decreasing the dosage usually relieves these complaints. Hypothyroidism may develop (particularly in women) during prolonged treatment. Isolated cases of reversible nephrogenic diabetes insipidus have been reported (Kudrow, 1980).

Summarizing his experience of more than 100 patients treated with lithium carbonate, Kudrow (1980) concludes the following.

1. Patients with the chronic type of cluster headache and those with more prolonged cluster periods in the episodic type respond best.

2. An average daily dose of 600mg and occasionally of 900mg suffices; this can be reduced to a maintenance dose of 300mg in about 10% of patients.

3. Ergotamine prophylaxis, combined with lithium, is required for complete relief of cluster headache by about 40% of patients.

4. After treatment with lithium is withdrawn, about 20% of patients whose chronic cluster headaches improved will have shorter episodic clusters.

The mode of action of lithium is unknown. It is postulated that its beneficial effect in cluster headache may be related to central regulation of cyclic biosynthesis and, indirectly, to vasomotor regulation.

Indomethacin

In Chapter 6 it was mentioned that treatment with indomethacin is dramatically effective for relief from daily, severe paroxysmal headaches in the very rare condition called "chronic paroxysmal hemicrania" by Sjaastad and Dale (1974). In his book *Cluster Headache,* Kudrow (1980) states that some patients with the chronic type of cluster headache also obtain relief from indomethacin. The drug would therefore merit a trial in a dose of 25mg three times daily for patients who have failed to respond to lithium, prednisone or methysergide. Gastrointestinal side effects to indomethacin are not uncommon and caution is necessary when prescribing it for patients with a history of peptic ulcer, epilepsy or psychiatric disorders.

Considering the episodic incidence, short duration and the extreme severity of pain in all types of cluster headache, prevention of attacks helps the patient more than symptomatic treatment once the headache has started.

The following approach to the prophylactic treatment of the two main varieties of cluster headache is recommended. It is based on the success of each drug in the author's experience of more than 60 cases and on reports published in the literature. The plan of action, therapeutic limitations, and side effects of the drugs prescribed must be carefully explained to the patient. They should keep records of the time, severity and duration of each attack and their progress must be reviewed frequently so that results can be assessed and the treatment strategy changed if the cluster headaches are not significantly controlled.

A. Episodic type of cluster headache

1. Start with methysergide, building the dose up gradually to 2mg three times daily. If this fails to prevent the attacks after a trial of 10 days, or if methysergide is not tolerated, replace it with the following.

2. Tablets containing a combination of 1mg to 2mg ergotamine tartrate with 100mg caffeine to be taken in the morning and evening. If orally administered ergotamine does not succeed after a trial of seven days, teach patients to administer to themselves a hypodermic or intramuscular injection of 0.5mg to 1.0mg dihydroergotamine mesylate in the morning and evening. The injections should be omitted for one day at the end of each week so that patients can determine when the cluster has come to its natural termination. For this prolonged treatment, the dose of orally administered ergotamine should not exceed 4mg in 24 hours and the dose of dihydroergotamine injections should not be greater than 2mg per 24 hours.

3. If both methysergide and ergotamine have failed to prevent the attacks, a course of treatment with prednisone or prednisolone in the doses outlined earlier in this chapter should be prescribed. Prednisone can be combined with oral ergotamine and caffeine, twice daily, or with self-administered injections of dihydroergotamine. A second course of treatment with corticosteroids can be prescribed after an interval of one week if the cluster headaches recur after completion of the first course.

4. If the above measures are not effective or not tolerated by the patient, lithium should be tried in doses ranging from 500mg to 1g per day. Lithium combined with ergotamines is sometimes the only successful treatment for patients over the age of 50 years.

B. Chronic type of cluster headache

1. Start with 250mg lithium carbonate morning and evening and increase gradually to 500mg every 12 hours if necessary. Alternately, the controlled release formulation of 800mg lithium carbonate can be taken in the morning or on going to bed. Further doses are determined from serum lithium levels, which should not exceed 1.2mmol/L. If some attacks of cluster headache continue, oral administrations of ergotamine tartrate with caffeine can be added once or twice daily.

2. If lithium does not prevent the headaches, it should be replaced with courses of prednisone or prednisolone in the doses previously outlined. Ergotamines can also be combined with corticosteroids. In view of the chronicity of this uncommon variety of cluster headache, the attacks are likely to recur once the steroids are withdrawn. Repeated courses of steroid therapy must be used with great caution, so that gastric erosions, cataracts, decalcification of bone, steroid myopathy and the other well known side effects of chronic corticosteroids do not develop. In the essential long intervals between courses of steroids small doses of ergotamines may make the patient's life more tolerable.

3. Indomethacin in a dose of 25mg three times a day is worth a trial if treatment with lithium and steroids fails.

Symptomatic Treatment for an Attack of Cluster Headache

The measures outlined above succeed in preventing attacks of cluster headache in from 65% to 85% of cases. The paroxysms will also continue during the initial period of trial before the most effective drug for prophylaxis in an individual patient has been determined.

The slow onset of action of analgesic drugs taken by mouth limits their use for severe headaches, which usually continue for only 60 to 90 minutes. Injections of narcotic analgesics must be avoided because of their potential for dependence or addiction. This leaves us with two measures, which were proven to have a good effect in a high proportion of patients.

1. Injections of 0.5mg to 1.0mg dihydroergotamine mesylate
As these are effective only at the onset of an attack, patients must learn to administer the injection themselves, or a relative living with the patient can be taught to give it. Parenterally administered ergotamine has a peak effect within two to 11 minutes and maintains its vasoconstrictor action for over two hours. Ergotamine is effective in the treatment of about 80% of attacks of cluster headache, but, in some instances, it fails completely to relieve the pain even if administered early. No explanation for such failures has been put forward.

2. Inhalation of 100% oxygen
Although reports of the success of oxygen inhalation in the treatment of cluster headache first appeared 30 years ago, this method of treatment has received increasing attention only in recent years. In a controlled study completed by 52 patients, 39 (75%) reported that 70% of all attacks were either aborted or reduced to a dull, tolerable pain within 15 minutes of oxygen inhalation. The oxygen is supplied from commercially available small oxygen cylinders with attached flow regulators. The patient inhales the gas through a loosely

applied facial mask at a rate of 7L to 8L per minute for a period of 15 minutes (Kudrow, 1980). It was found that males under the age of 50 years with the episodic type of cluster headache achieved the best responses to oxygen inhalation (80.8%), whereas patients over the age of 50 years with the chronic variety of the disease obtained relief in only 57.1% of cases.

The mechanism of action of oxygen in cluster headache is unknown. Sakai and Meyer (1979) were able to show that the administration of 100% oxygen rapidly reduced cerebral blood flow during the attack. Therefore, it may be assumed that the increased cerebral blood flow, more marked on the side contralateral to the headache during the attack, is in some way implicated in the mechanism of pain production.

Oxygen inhalation has the advantage of having no adverse side effects. When this treatment modality is considered, it is advisable to admit the patient to hospital for a few days during a cluster to test the effect of oxygen. If it succeeds, the patient can rent oxygen cylinders and regulators and continue treating himself at home until the end of the cluster. If necessary, ergotamine by the oral, rectal or parenteral route can be used in combination with oxygen inhalation, and the patient will have to rely on oral, sublingual or inhalant ergotamine preparations for attacks which occur away from home.

Surgical Treatment of Cluster Headache

As the pain of cluster headache is so intense, it is not surprising that a variety of surgical approaches have been tried on patients who had failed to improve with medical treatment. These include: (i) avulsion or alcohol block of the supraorbital nerve; (ii) section of the ophthalmic division of the trigeminal nerve or of the greater superficial petrosal nerve; and (iii) section of the nervus intermedius to interrupt the proximal parasympathetic outflow to the petrosal nerves. Cryosurgical (freezing) techniques were applied more recently to the sphenopalatine ganglion and to the superficial temporal and occipital arteries. The small number of patients subjected to the earlier operations and the short periods of follow-up do not permit valid conclusions about the success of these procedures. Cryosurgical techniques had limited success in patients with episodic cluster headache with short remissions and in a few chronic cases. The recurrence rate was high and about one-third of patients complained of persistent numbness of the face on the operated side (Kudrow, 1980). At the present time, surgery should be considered only for the few, isolated people who have intolerable pain which has proved refractory to an adequate trial of all non-surgical treatment modalities.

Surgical Treatment of Migraine

Surgical endeavours to relieve migrainous hemicrania date from the beginning of this century because the pharmaceutical remedies available at that time had not met with much success. In a review of the history of the surgeons' approaches to migraine, Knight (1968) describes the pathogenetic assumptions on which these operations were based. It is interesting that some of the foremost neurosurgeons of their era, including Adson, Dandy, Olivecrona and Penfield published papers on the rationale, technique and success of their operations. These papers dealt with only a small number of cases, with short and often inadequate follow-up observations, and the results were not very satisfactory. The dearth of literature on new and better surgical procedures during the past 15 years indicates that surgery has a very small place in the treatment of migraine and its variants.

The earliest operations were directed at the cervical part of the sympathetic nervous system and were motivated by the erroneous premise that the first phase of cerebral vasoconstriction actually *caused* the subsequent painful dilation of cranial vessels. Therefore, cervical sympathectomy or excision of the stellate ganglion was performed to prevent cerebral angiospasm. Some 20 years later, other surgeons modified the technique to a periarterial sympathectomy of the carotid bifurcation combined with excision of the superior cervical ganglion and ligature and division of the external carotid artery. Knight (1968) points out that the rich anastomotic circulation in the scalp would quickly counteract any beneficial result from external carotid ligation. He restricted his operations to stripping the periarterial sympathetic plexus from the carotid bifurcation combined with superior cervical ganglionectomy. He thought that this operation would favourably influence cerebral angiospastic phenomena such as hemiparaesthesia, dysphasia and transient pareses, as well as hemicranial headaches. In a series of 12 unilateral operations, three patients obtained complete relief, seven enjoyed some reduction in the frequency and severity of headaches and two operations were complete failures. Unfortunately, the period of follow-up observation is not stated.

When it was found that relief from vascular headache could not be achieved from interruption of the sympathetic pathways, surgeons turned their attention to the afferent pain fibres in the trigeminal nerve and its central connections. The anatomical course of afferent nerves from cranial vessels is not definitely established. It is thought that some fibres from the carotid plexus may reach the brain stem via the nervus intermedius. The supraorbital and frontal branches of the ophthalmic artery and the superficial temporal artery are supplied by branches of the trigeminal nerve. Pain arising in occipital and suboccipital scalp vessels is conducted centrally through posterior auricular and great occipital nerves to the upper cervical sensory nerve roots.

Operations were performed at every level of these anatomical pathways. The operations ranged from section of cutaneous nerves such as the supraorbital and auriculotemporal branches of the trigeminus, and section of the great occipital and posterior auricular nerves, to alcohol injection of the trigeminal (Gasserian) ganglion and fractional section of the trigeminal sensory root. Even medullary tractotomy, where pain fibres in the descending (spinal) tract of the trigeminal nerve are destroyed, was experimented with. All these operations were, of course, reserved for the most severe and intractable cases. The results were generally disappointing and most patients were left with a feeling of numbness and with unpleasant dysaesthesia on one side of the face and forehead, while the headaches continued. The only procedure which would still justify consideration in patients with exceptionally severe pain which remains unrelieved by all other therapeutic modalities is radiofrequency coagulation of the trigeminal ganglion. It is a relatively simple surgical procedure, but very painful as it can be performed only with local anaesthesia. The patient has to be warned that the face on the side of the pain will become numb, but this is usually tolerable when the operation is performed for relief from trigeminal neuralgia. The opinions of other neurologists and neurosurgeons should be obtained before a person, desperate with intractable headache, is subjected to radiofrequency coagulation. As any surgical procedure can be considered only for hemicrania which has been consistently on the same side for months or years patients must be told that a similar pain can still occur on the opposite side after a successful operation.

As distension of branches of the external carotid artery contributes to the pathogenetic mechanisms of vascular headache of migraine type, ligation or division of the external carotid artery, or of its branches, has been performed in carefully selected cases. Earlier experience had shown that ligation of the middle meningeal vessels or of the common carotid artery failed to relieve hemicrania. Common carotid ligation also involves the patient in the risk of ischaemia in an internal carotid distribution — a risk which is not justified in the treatment of migraine, however severe. The extensive crosscirculation in the scalp would make any lasting beneficial effect from ligation of the common or external carotid artery very unlikely. However, this consideration would not apply to the same extent to ligation of the superficial temporal artery or of other branches of the external carotid. Such operations could be expected to provide relief only in the very rare instances where headache is consistently localized to the area of distribution of a particular branch of the external carotid. Even then, it is possible that headache will recur in a different area or on the opposite side. Holland (1976) described two cases where migrainous headaches were felt only in the region of one superficial temporal artery and were temporarily relieved by pressure applied to this vessel. The headache appeared after a minor injury to the temple in one patient and after a tantalum cranioplasty in the other. Whereas the commonly used prophylactic agents and injections of ergotamine provided no or at best partial relief, the headaches ceased completely after superficial temporal artery ligation during a one to two year follow-up observation of these patients. The onset of strictly localized vascular headache after trauma in these patients justified the trial of ligation of a branch of the external carotid artery, which proved successful. The history of trauma reduced the probability of recurrence on the other side. The patients' repeated observations that compression of the artery abolished pain for a short period suggested that headache arose from distension of this vessel.

This brief review of surgical endeavours in the treatment of migraine may help the primary physician to explain to patients, disappointed by the failure of drug therapy, that no operations are available to ease their pain. The cases where pain remains localized to the territory of a single branch of the external carotid artery are the only and rare exceptions to this rule.

Summary of Management of Patients with Migraine

1. Infrequent attacks at irregular intervals

Treat the attack with metoclopramide and aspirin or ergotamines during the aura or at the onset of headache.

2. Frequency of attacks averaging 12 to 18 per year

A. Determine the triggers of the attacks and try to avoid or manipulate them.

B. Assess the patient's personality profile. If the patient is tense or unable to relax try hypnosis, relaxation training and/or biofeedback. Short courses of minor tranquillizers may be of assistance.

C. Restrict drug therapy to times or situations of high risk of attacks. Prophylactic drugs should be changed only after adequate trial of the maximum tolerated dose or if side effects occur. Start treatment with propranolol and, if necessary, change to: pizotifen; then Bellergal; then cyproheptadine or methdilazine.

3. Frequency of attacks averaging more than 18 per year

A. Identify and avoid or manipulate trigger factors.

B. Counselling and hypnosis may be of aid, then relaxation training and/or biofeedback, if the patient's anxious personality contributes to migraine.

C. Follow this with sustained prophylactic drug treatment with propranolol or pizotifen as drugs of first choice. If these are not effective, or are badly tolerated, change to Bellergal and finally to methysergide (with due precautions); particularly if the condition is classic migraine and headaches are severe. If all else fails, phenelzine may be tried.

4. Management of acute attack

A. Drug administration during aura or at the onset of headache is essential.

B. If the patient does not feel bilious, start treatment with oral metoclopramide and a large dose of soluble aspirin. If this fails, replace the aspirin with a compound preparation of ergotamine and caffeine with or without antihistamine. Repeat administration of this preparation after one to two hours if necessary.

C. If nausea occurs early in the attack and if circumstances permit, try using a Cafergot suppository and a prochlorperazine suppository; if this treatment fails, treat the next attack with injections of metoclopramide and dihydroergotamine. These can be repeated after an hour.

D. If a moderate headache continues, administer compound tablets of aspirin or paracetamol with codeine later in the attack.

E. If severe headache and vomiting continue, injections of narcotic analgesics and metoclopramide, prochlorperazine or thiethylperazine are the best treatment.

5. Management of status migrainosus.

A. Heavy sedation in an attempt to keep patient asleep for prolonged periods. If this fails try the following.

B. Prescribe a course of corticosteroids such as prednisone or dexamethasone.

C. If status migrainosus is severe and prolonged, admit the patient to hospital.

Chapter 8

Epilogue

Although the clinical features of migraine were known for more than 2000 years and Liveing provided a good acount of the disease in 1873, concepts of aetiology and treatment were still rather chaotic at the beginning of this century. During the past 50 years, some order was brought into this chaos and advances in knowledge have accelerated since 1960. We now have a clear definition of the many variants included in the broad concept of migraine, we have established its multifactorial aetiology, and we are beginning to understand some of the physiological and biochemical changes which play a part in its pathogenesis. The last two decades have seen a more scientific approach to the treatment of migraine and controlled trials of any drug or non-pharmaceutical therapeutic approach are demanded before the success of treatment is accepted. As complete cure, in the proper sense of this word, remains an unattainable goal, some patients and physicians are still drawn to the unscientific superstitions of "alternative medicine" in their search for relief.

Of course, it is true that there is a lot more to learn about the causes and treatment of migraine. Our knowledge of the role of amines, prostaglandins and bradykinin is only fragmentary and new horizons are opening with the discovery of neuropeptides in the brain, which appear to be involved in the feeling of pain. We have sound physiological evidence for intracranial vasoconstriction and extracranial vasodilation, but still remain ignorant as to why these changes in vascular calibre can be localized to specific regions of the brain or scalp, which may change from attack to attack.

From the knowledge we have acquired we may assume that a person is born with a propensity to migraine and this may be determined by anomalies in platelet aggregability or in central or peripheral serotonergic function. Such people will react to changes in the external or internal environment with an attack of common or classic migraine, whereas their non-migrainous fellows can deal with the same events without developing symptoms. The physician cannot change the constitution of migraineurs, but can help them to discover and avoid some of the offending triggers. We can teach some of our patients to relax and, with the aid of modern technology, can prove to them that their headaches, however severe, are not due to some sinister and progressive mischief within their cranium.

In the vast majority of patients we are able to alleviate the severe headache and associated gastrointestinal disorders, but it takes patience and time to discover the best remedies for each individual person. We should inform our patients that we cannot hope for complete cure, but that the treatment recommended will markedly reduce the frequency and severity of their attacks. In this regard, migraine does not differ significantly from other paroxysmal disorders, such as epilepsy or asthma, or from many of the common diseases of the cardiovascular, alimentary or respiratory systems. As in all branches of medicine, a small hard core of intractable cases will always remain.

The advent of special societies for the study of migraine in several countries, the large volume of research into every aspect of the disease throughout the world, and the efficient means of communication among scientists justify an optimistic outlook for the future. During the next decade, better drugs for the prevention and treatment of vascular headache of migraine type should become available. We can tell our patients that the prognosis for greater relief, if not for cure, is good.

References

Ad Hoc Committee on Classification of Headache of the National Institute of Neurological Diseases and Blindness: Classification of headache. Journal of the American Medical Association 179: 717-718 (1962).

Aellig, W.H. and Nuesch, E.: Comparative pharmaco-kinetic investigations with tritium-labelled ergot alkaloids after oral and intravenous administration in man. International Journal of Clinical Pharmacology 15: 106-111 (1977).

Ala-Hurula, V.; Myllylä, V.V.; Arvela, P.; Heikkilä, J.; Kärki, N. and Hokkanen, E.: Systemic availability of ergotamine tartrate after oral, rectal and intramuscular administration. European Journal of Clinical Pharmacology 15: 51-55 (1979).

American Hospital Formulary Service. Ergotamine tartrate. Sympatholytic agents 12: 16 (1981).

Anderson, J.A.D.; Basker, M.A. and Dalton, R.: Migraine and hypnotherapy. International Journal of Clinical and Experimental Hypnosis 23: 48-58 (1975).

Andreychuk, T. and Skriver, C.: Hypnosis and biofeedback in the treatment of migraine headache. International Journal of Clinical and Experimental Hypnosis 23: 172-183 (1975).

Anthony, M.: The mechanisms underlying migraine. Medical Journal of Australia 2 (Suppl): 11-15 (1972a).

Anthony, M.: Migrainous neuralgia — an allergic disorder? Hemicrania 4/3: 2-5 (1972b).

Anthony, M.: Individual free fatty acids and migraine. Clinical and Experimental Neurology (Proceedings of the Australian Association of Neurologists) 15: 190-196 (1978).

Anthony, M. and Hinterberger, H.: Amine turnover in migraine. Proceedings of the Australian Association of Neurologists 12: 43-47 (1975).

Anthony, M. and Lance, J.W.: Monoamine oxidase inhibition in the treatment of migraine. Archives of Neurology 21: 263-268 (1969).

Anthony, M. and Lance, J.W.: Histamine and serotonin in cluster headache. Archives of Neurology 25: 225-231 (1971).

Anthony, M.; Lance, J.W. and Lord, G.: Migrainous neuralgia — Blood histamine levels and clinical response to H_1 and H_2 receptor blockade; in Green (Ed) Current Concepts in Migraine Research, p. 149-151 (Raven Press, New York, 1978).

Balla, J.I. and Walton, J.N.: Periodic migrainous neuralgia. British Medical Journal 1: 219-221 (1964).

Balyeat, R.M. and Rinkel, H.J.: Allergic migraine in children. Americal Journal of Diseases in Children 42: 1126-1133 (1931).

Barolin, G.S.: Migräne, p 43 (Facultas-Verlag, Wien, 1969).

Barolin, G.S.: Bioelectric findings and migraines; in Dalessio, Dalsgaard-Nielsen and Diamond (Eds) Proceedings of the International Headache Symposium, p. 9-21 (Sandoz, Basle, 1971).

Basser, L.S.: The relation of migraine and epilepsy. Brain 92/2: 285-300 (1969).

Bickerstaff, E.R.: Basilar artery migraine. Lancet 1: 15-17 (1961).

Bickerstaff, E.R.: The basilar artery and the migraine-epilepsy syndrome. Proceedings of the Royal Society of Medicine 55: 167-169 (1962).

Bille, B.: Migraine in school children. Acta Paediatrica Scandinavica 51 (Suppl) 136: 1-151 (1962).

Bille, B.: Headaches in children; in Vinken and Bruyn (Eds) Handbook of Clinical Neurology, vol. 5, p. 239-246 (North-Holland Publishing Company, Amsterdam, 1968).

Blau, J.N. and Whitty, C.W.M.: Familial hemiplegic migraine. Lancet 2: 1115-1116 (1955).

Bogduk, N.: Headaches and cervical manipulation. Medical Journal of Australia 2: 65-66 (1979).

Bradshaw, P. and Parsons, M.: Hemiplegic migraine, a clinical study. Quarterley Journal of Medicine 34: 65-85 (1965).

Brewis, M.; Poskanzer, D.C.; Rolland, C. and Miller, H.: Neurological disease in an English city. Acta Neurologica Scandinavica 42: Suppl. 24 (1966).

Bruyn, G.W.: Complicated migraine; in Vinken and Bruyn (Eds) Handbook of Clinical Neurology, vol 5, p. 59-95 (North-Holland Publishing Company, Amsterdam, 1968).

Bruyn, G.W. and Gathier, J.C.: Migraine and Methysergide. An appraisal. Proceedings of the Australian Association of Neurologists 5/3: 643-649 (1968).

Cala, L.A. and Mastaglia, F.L.: Computerized axial tomography findings in a group of patients with migrainous headaches. Proceedings of the Australian Association of Neurologists 13: 35-41 (1976).

Cala, L.A. and Mastaglia, F.L.: Computerized axial tomography in the detection of brain damage. 2. Eilepsy, migraine and general medical disorders. Medical Journal of Australia 2: 616-620 (1980).

Chapman, L.F.; Ramos, A.O.; Goodell, H.; Silverman, G. and Wolff, H.G.: A humoral agent implicated in vascular headache of the migraine type. Archives of Neurology 3: 223-229 (1960).

Childs, A.J. and Sweetnam, M.T.: A study of 104 cases of migraine. British Journal of Industrial Medicine 18: 234-236 (1961).

Couch, J.R.; Ziegler, D.K. and Hassanein, R.: Amitriptyline in the prophylaxis of migraine. Neurology 26: 121-127 (1976).

Curran, D.A.; Hinterberger, H. and Lance, J.W.: Total plasma serotonin, 5-hydroxyindoleacetic acid and p-hydroxy-m-methoxy-mandelic acid excretion in normal and migrainous subjects. Brain 88: 997-1010 (1965).

Dalessio, D.J.: Headache mechanisms; in Vinken and Bruyn (Eds) Handbook of Clinical Neurology, vol. 5, p. 15-16 (North-Holland Publishing Company, Amsterdam, 1968).

Dalessio, D.J.: Some current data on headache research. Triangle, Sandoz Journal of Medical Science 20 (1/2): 33-41 (1981).

Dalsgaard-Nielsen, T.: Migraine and heredity. Acta Neurologica Scandinavica 41: 287-300 (1965).

de la Lande, I.S.; Cannell, V.A. and Waterson, J.G.: The interaction of serotonin and noradrenaline on the perfused artery. British Journal of Pharmacology 28: 255-272 (1966).

Diamond, S. and Medina, J.L.: Double-blind study of propranolol for migraine prophylaxis. Headache 16 (1): 24-27 (1976).

Dorfman, L.J.; Marshall, W.H. and Enzmann, D.R.: Cerebral infarction and migraine: Clinical and radiologic correlations. Neurology 29: 317-322 (1979).

Dow, D.J. and Whitty, C.W.M.: Electroencephalographic changes in migraine. Review of 51 cases. Lancet 261: 52-54 (1947).

Eadie, M.J.; Sutherland, J.M. and Tyrer, J.H.: Recurrent monocular blindness of uncertain cause. Lancet 1: 319-321 (1968).

Eadie, M.J. and Tyrer, J.H.: Migraine; in Neurological Clinical Pharmacology, p. 255-284 (Adis Press, Sydney, 1980).

Ekbom, K.A.: Ergotamine tartrate orally in Horton's "histaminic cephalgia" (also called Harris's "ciliary neuralgia"). A new method of treatment. Acta Psychiatrica Scandinavica (Suppl) 46: 106-113 (1947).

Ekbom, K.: A clinical comparison of cluster headache and migraine. Acta Neurologica Scandinavica 46: Suppl. 41 (1970).

Ekbom, K.: Litium vid kroniska symptom av cluster headache. Preliminärt Meddelande. Pousc. Med. 19: 148-156 (1974) (cited by Kudrow, 1980).

Fanchamps, A.: Sandoz — Fifty years' involvement in migraine therapy. Triangle 15: 103-110 (1976).

Fozard, J.R. and Schnieden, H.: Factors affecting the control and reactivity of blood vessels. Hemicrania 4/2: 3-7 (1972).

Friedman, A.P.; Migraine. Pathophysiology and pathogenesis; in Vinken and Bruyn (Eds) Handbook of Clinical Neurology, vol. 5, p. 37-44 (North-Holland Publishing Company, Amsterdam, 1968).

Friedman, A.P.; Harter D.H. and Merritt, H.H.: Ophthalmoplegic migraine. Archives of Neurology 7: 320-327 (1962).

Friedman, A.P. and Mikropolos, H.E.: Cluster headaches. Neurology 8: 653-663 (1958).

Friedman, A.P.: Von Storch, T.C.J. and Merritt, H.H.: Migraine and tension headache: a clinical study of two thousand cases. Neurology 4: 733-788 (1954).

Friedman, H. and Taub, H.A.: An evaluation of hypnotic susceptibility and peripheral temperature elevation in the treatment of migraine. American Journal of Clinical Hypnosis 24: 172-182 (1982).

Gowers, W.R.: A Manual of Diseases of the Nervous System, p. 836-856 (P. Blakiston, Son & Co., Philadelphia, 1893).

Graham, J.R.: Cardiac and pulmonary fibrosis during methysergide therapy for headache. American Journal of Medical Sciences 254: 23-34 (1967).

Graham, J.R.: Migraine. Clinical aspects; in Vinken and Bruyn (Eds) Handbook of Clinical Neurology, vol. 5, p. 45-58 (North-Holland Publishing Company, Amsterdam, 1968).

Graham, J.R. and Wolff, H.G.: Mechanism of migraine headache and action of ergotamine tartrate. Archives of Neurology and Psychiatry 39: 737-763 (1938).

Greene, R.: Water retention in migraine. Proceedings of the Royal Society of Medicine 55: 169-171 (1962).

Hanington, E.: Migraine. A platelet hypothesis. Biomedicine 30: 65-66 (1979).

Harris, W.: Neuritis and Neuralgia, p. 145-146, 301-313 (Oxford University Press, Oxford, 1926).

Harris, W.: Ciliary (migrainous) neuralgia and its treatment. British Medical Journal 1: 457-460 (1936).

Heathfield, K.W.G. and Raiman, J.D.: An open evaluation of dixarit in four hospitals; in Proceedings of Cambridge Symposium on the Migraine Headache and Dixarit, p. 16-23 (Boehringer Ingelheim, Bracknell, 1972).

Heyck, H.: Neue Beiträge zur Klinik und Pathogenese der Migräne, p. 65-69 (Georg Thieme Verlag, Stuttgart, 1956).

Heyck, H.: Der Kopfschmerz. Differentialdiagnostik und Therapie für die Praxis, p. 49-50, 62-70 (Georg Thieme Verlag, Stuttgart, 1958).

Hilton, B.P.: Blood platelets: a pathological difference between migrainous and control subjects. Hemicrania 3/2: 3-5 (1971).

Hinrichs, W.L. and Keith, H.M.: Migraine in childhood: A follow-up report. Mayo Clinic Proceedings 40: 593-596 (1965).

Holland, J.T.: Three cases of post traumatic vascular headache treated by surgery. Proceedings of the Australian Association of Neurologists 13: 51-54 (1976).

Horton, B.T.: The use of histamine in the treatment of specific types of headache. Journal of the American Medical Association 116: 377-383 (1941).

Horton, B.T.: Histaminic cephalgia. Differential diagnosis and treatment: 1176 patients 1937-1955. Proceedings of Staff Meetings of the Mayo Clinic 31: 325-333 (1956).

Hungerford, G.D.; du Boulay, G.H. and Zilkha, K.J.: Computerized axial tomography in patients with severe migraine: A preliminary report. Journal of Neurology, Neurosurgery and Psychiatry 39: 990-994 (1976).

Jammes, J.L.: The treatment of cluster headache with prednisone. Diseases of the Nervous System 36: 375-376 (1975).

Kallós, P. and Kallós-Deffner, L.: Allergy and migraine. International Archives of Allergy 7: 367-372 (1955).

Kim, S.S.: Acupuncture: mode of action in migraine headache. American Journal of Acupuncture 3/2: 108-114 (1975).

Klee, A.: A clinical study of migraine with particular reference to the most severe cases (Munksgaard, Copenhagen, 1968).

Knight, G.: Surgical treatment of migraine: in Vinken and Bruyn (Eds) Handbook of Clinical Neurology, vol. 5, p. 104-110 (North-Holland Publishing Company, Amsterdam, 1968).

Krayenbühl, H. and Heyck, H.: The prophylactic treatment of migraine. International Archives of Allergy 7: 339-347 (1955).

Kudrow, L.: Lithium prophylaxis for chronic cluster headache. Headache 17: 15-18 (1977).

Kudrow L.: Comparative results of prednisone, methysergide, and lithium therapy in cluster headache; in Greene (Ed) Current Concepts in Migraine Research, p. 159-163 (Raven Press, New York, 1978).

Kudrow, L.: Cluster Headache. Mechanisms and Management, p. 127-154 (Oxford University Press, New York, 1980).

Kudrow, L. and Sutkus, B.J.: MMPI pattern specificity in primary headache disorders. Headache 19: 18-24 (1979).

Kunkle, E.C.; Pfeiffer, J.P.; Wilhoit, W.M. and Hamrick, L.W.: Recurrent brief headache in "cluster" pattern. Transactions of the American Neurological Association 77: 240-243 (1952).

Lance, J.W.: Leading article. Hemicrania 2/4: 4-8 (1970).

Lance, J.W.: Clinical features and vascular changes of migraine and cluster headache. Medical Journal of Australia (Suppl) 2: 3-6 (1972a).

Lance, J.W.: Interval therapy in migraine. Medical Journal of Australia (Suppl) 2: 29-32 (1972b).

Lance, J.W.: Headaches related to sexual activity. Journal of Neurology, Neurosurgery and Psychiatry 39: 1226-1230 (1976).

Lance, J.W. and Anthony, M.: Some clinical aspects of migraine. Archives of Neurology 15: 356-361 (1966).

Lance, J.W. and Anthony, M.: Thermographic studies in vascular headache. Medical Journal of Australia 1: 240-243 (1971).

Lance, J.W.; Anthony, M. and Somerville, B.: Comparative trial of serotonin antagonists in the management of migraine. British Medical Journal 2: 327-330 (1970).

Leão, A.A.P.: Spreading depression of activity in cerebral cortex. Journal of Neurophysiology 7: 359-390 (1944).

Liveing, E.: On Megrim, Sick-Headache and Some Allied Disorders: A Contribution to the Pathology of Nerve-Storms (Churchill, London, 1873).

Lundberg, P.O.: Abdominal migraine. Triangle 17/2: 81-84 (1978).

Matthews, W.B.: Footballer's migraine. British Medical Journal 2/5809: 326-327 (1972).

Mazal, S. and Rachmilewitz, E.A.: The effect of an antiserotonin agent pizotifen on platelet aggregability in migraine patients. Journal of Neurology, Neurosurgery and Psychiatry 43: 1137-1140 (1980).

McHenry, L.C.Jr.: Garrison's History of Neurology, p. 398-400 (Charles C. Thomas, Springfield, 1969).

Monro, J.; Brostoff, J.; Carini, C. and Zilkha, K.: Food allergy in migraine: Study of dietary exclusion and RAST. Lancet 2: 1-4 (1980).

Moser, M.; Wish, H. and Friedman, A.P.: Headache and hypertension. Journal of the American Medical Association 180: 301-306 (1962).

O'Brien, M.D.: Cerebral blood changes in migraine. Headache 10/4: 139-143 (1971).

Office of Health Economics. Prevalence and incidence of migraine; in "Migraine" No. 41, p. 7-12 (Office of Health Economics, London, 1972).

O'Neill, B.P. and Mann, J.D.: Aspirin prophylaxis in migraine. Lancet 2: 1179-1181 (1978).

Parker, G.B.; Tupling, H. and Pryor, D.S.: A controlled trial of cervical manipulation for migraine. Australian and New Zealand Journal of Medicine 8: 589-593 (1978).

Pearce, J.M.S.: Chronic migrainous neuralgia. A variant of cluster headache. Brain 103: 149-159 (1980).

Prensky, A.L. and Sommer, D.: Diagnosis and treatment of migraine in children. Neurology 29: 506-510 (1979).

Raskin, N.H.: Pharmacology of migraine. Annual Reviews of Pharmacology and Toxicology 21: 463-478 (1981).

Refsum, S.: Genetic aspects of migraine; in Vinken and Bruyn (Eds) Handbook of Clinical Neurology, vol. 5, p. 258-259 (North-Holland Publishing Company, Amsterdam, 1968).

Research Group on Migraine and Headache of the World Federation of Neurology. Definition of Migraine. Hemicrania 1/1: 3 (1969).

Sacks, O.W.: Migraine. The Evolution of a Common Disorder. (Faber and Faber Ltd., London, 1971).

Sakai, F. and Meyer, J.S.: Abnormal cerebrovascular reactivity in patients with migraine and cluster headache. Headache 19: 257-266 (1979).

Sandler, M.: Youdim, M.B.H. and Hanington, E.: A phenylethylamine oxidising defect in migraine. Nature 250/5464: 335-337 (1974).

Sargent, J.D.; Walters, E.D. and Green, E.E.: Psychosomatic self-regulation of migraine headaches. Seminars in Psychiatry 5/4: 415-428 (1973).

Selby, G.: A clinical trial of an antiserotonin drug, BC-105, in the prophylaxis of migraine. Proceedings of the Australian Association of Neurologists 7: 37-43 (1970).

Selby, G. and Lance, J.W.: Observations on 500 cases of migraine and allied vascular headache. Journal of Neurology, Neurosurgery and Psychiatry 23: 23-32 (1960).

Sicuteri, F.: Franchi, G. and Del Bianco, P.L.: An antaminic drug, BC 105, in the prophylaxis of migraine. International Archives of Allergy 31: 78-93 (1967).

Sicuteri, F.; Testi, A. and Anselmi, B.: Biochemical investigations in headache: Increase in hydroxyindole-acetic acid excretion during migraine attacks. International Archives of Allergy 19: 55-58 (1961).

Shaw, D.A. and Saunders, M.: A double-blind comparison of dixarit and placebo; in Proceedings of Cambridge Symposium on the Migraine Headache and Dixarit, p. 54-61 (Boehringer Ingelheim, Bracknell, 1972).

Sjaastad, O. and Dale, I.: Evidence for a new (?) treatable headache entity. Headache 14: 105-108 (1974).

Skinhøj, E.: The value of regional blood flow studies in migraine research; in Background to Migraine, Sixth Migraine Symposium, p. 3 (Migraine Trust, London, 1974).

Slatter, K.H.: Some clinical and EEG findings in patients with migraine. Brain 91: 85-98 (1968).

Smith, I.; Kellow, A.H. and Hanington, E.: A clinical and biochemical correlation between tyramine and migraine headache. Headache 10/2: 43-52 (1970).

Smyth, V.O.G. and Winter, A.L.: The EEG in migraine. Electroencephalography and Clinical Neurophysiology 16: 194-202 (1964).

Somerville, B.W.: The role of estradiol withdrawal in the etiology of menstrual migraine. Neurology 22/4: 355-365 (1972a).

Somerville, B.W.: A study of migraine in pregnancy. Neurology 22/8: 824-828 (1972b).

Somerville, B.W.: Migraine: The serotonin theory re-examined. Hemicrania 7/3: 2-5 (1976).

Sutherland, J.M. and Eadie, M.J.: Cluster headache; in Research and Clinical Studies in Headache, vol. 3, p. 92-125 (Karger, Basle, 1972).

Sutherland, J.M.; Hooper, W.D.; Eadie, M.J. and Tyrer, J.H.: Buccal absorption of ergotamine. Journal of Neurology, Neurosurgery and Psychiatry 37: 1116-1120 (1974).

Symonds, C.P.: Migrainous variants. Transactions of the Medical Society of London 67: 237-251 (1951).

Symonds, C.P.: A particular variety of headache. Brain 79: 217-232 (1956a).

Symonds, C.P.: Cough headache. Brain 79: 557-568 (1956b).

Tallett, E.: A comprehensive study of dixarit: in Proceedings of Cambridge Symposium on the Migraine Headache and Dixarit, p. 77-85 (Boehringer Ingelheim, Bracknell, 1972).

Tork, I.: Innervation of cortical vessels. Neuro-science Letters (Suppl) 8: S 19 (1982).

Vahlquist, B.: Migraine in children. International Archives of Allergy 7: 348-355 (1955).

Walker, C.H.: Migraine and its relationship to hypertension. British Medical Journal 2: 1430-1433 (1959).

Walsh, F.B. and Hoyt, W.F.: Migraine; in Clinical Neuro-ophthalmology, 3rd ed. vol. 2, p. 1654-1689 (Williams and Wilkins Company, Baltimore, 1969).

Waters, W.E.: Migraine: Intelligence, social class and familial prevalence. British Medical Journal 2: 77-81 (1971).

Waters, W.E.: Migraine and symptoms in childhood: Bilious attacks, travel sickness and eczema. Headache 12/2: 55-61 (1972).

Weil, A.A.: EEG findings in a certain type of psychosomatic headache: Dysrhythmic migraine. Electroencephalography and Clinical Neurophysiology 4: 181-186 (1952).

Whisnant, J.P.: Personal communication. (1982).

Whitty, C.W.M.: Migraine and epilepsy. Hemicrania 4/1: 2-4 (1972).

Widerøe, T.E. and Vigander, T.: Propranolol in the treatment of migraine. British Medical Journal 2: 699-701 (1974).

Wilson, S.A. Kinnier: Neurology, A.N. Bruce (Ed), vol. 2, p. 1571-1572 (Edward Arnold & Co., London, 1940).

Wolff, H.G.: Headache and Other Head Pain, p. 386-387 (Oxford University Press, New York, 1963).

Subject Index

definition and classification 2-3
economic effect of 3, 4-5
equivalents of 67-72
origin of term 1-2
prevalence and incidence of 3-5
without headache 58-60, 80, 102-105
Migraine accompagnée 2, 37
Migraine syncope 3, 17, 35, 44, 106
Migrainous neuralgia 2
Migral 78
Monoamine oxidase enzymes 9, 10, 24, 25, 26
inhibitors of 98, 116-117
Monosodium glutamate 9
Motion sickness 15, 32
Movement disorders 41-42, 92, 105

N

Naproxen 115
Nausea 35, 45, 51 (case), 60, 61, 65, 94, 102, 104, 112, 113, 123
Neurokinin 24, 27
Neurological examination 74-81
Nicotinic acid 10
Nitroglycerine 63
Noradrenaline 24, 25, 26, 27, 28, 109, 116
Nuclear brain scans 82
Numbness 40, 41

O

Obsessional behaviour 8
Oestradiol valerate 12
Onions 9
Ophthalmological examinations 93, 104
Ophthalmoplegic migraine 2, 49-50, 51, 57, 105
Oral contraceptives 13, 120
Oranges 9
Oxygen 138-139

P

Paget's disease 71
Pain 21, 24, 60, 63, 64, 65, 98, 102
abdominal 69
Paraesthesia 36, 41, 42 (case), 45 (case), 46, 52, 55 (case), 71, 104, 105

Paresis 42, 49
Parry 1
Pathogenesis 20-30
Personality factors 7-8, 11, 75, 114
Phenelzine 116, 117, 118
Phenobarbitone 108, 109, 118
Phenylethylamine 9, 10, 27
Phenytoin 56, 118
Photophobia 34, 42 (case), 51 (case), 52 (case), 55 (case), 60, 61, 65, 66 (case), 73, 74, 100, 102
Pizotifen 26, 102, 110, 112, 114, 117, 135
Platelet hypothesis 24
Polypeptides 25, 27
Polyuria 34
Prednisone 67, 135, 137
Pregnancy 12, 35, 46, 110
Premenstrual syndrome 12-13
Primidone 56
Prochlorperazine maleate 118, 123
Progesterone 28
Propranolol 109-111, 114, 117, 118, 123
Prostaglandins 25, 28, 29, 30, 102, 115, 126, 143
inhibitors of synthesis 115-116
Psychological factors 7-8, 55

Q

Questionnaire 77-79

R

Radioallergosorbent tests 119
Red wine 10, 32, 117, 119
Relaxation 11, 32
training for 121-125
Reserpine 10, 25
Retinal symptoms 20
Rhinitis 17, 18, 112

S

Seizures 43, 53 (case), 92
Sensory symptoms 40-42
Serotonin 18, 24, 25-26, 27, 28, 29, 30, 63, 96, 108, 109, 111, 112, 113, 115, 126
Serum levels 93
Sex incidence 3, 4, 62